THE

7

STEPS

TO
OVERCOMING
DEPRESSION
AND
ANXIETY

THE
7
STEPS
TO
OVERCOMING
DEPRESSION
AND
ANXIETY

By
Gary Null

ibooks
new york
www.ibooks.net
DISTRIBUTED BY SIMON & SCHUSTER, INC.

Contents

Acknowledgements

Gary Null would like to thank the following people for
their contributions to the book:

Bob Dean

Andre Turan

Chef Marcus Guiliano,
for his culinary expertise

Dr. Dorothy Smith

and Lois Zinn

THE
7
STEPS
TO
OVERCOMING
DEPRESSION
AND
ANXIETY

INTRODUCTION

TODAY it would be easier to ask who is not depressed or anxious than who is. After all, look at the environment in which we live. 9/11 gave every American reason for concern with the government approval of terrorist insurance for future catastrophic events, nonstop reporting on "weapons of mass destruction" and the high probability of a war with Iraq. People now think twice before planning a vacation, wondering whether their plane will be shot down or their destination targeted by terrorists. More than ever, we are cognizant of our own vulnerability, aware that, in a second, our lives could end.

People are also anxious or depressed about the effects of an unstable economy. We have approximately six million millionaires, mostly upper mobile baby boomers. That seems great. But we also have more than 60 million people who are living at or below the level of the lower middle class who have less disposable income today than they did 25 years ago. We grew up believing that America is a land of opportunity, but it no longer seems to be that way. The middle class was told that, as long as they worked for one corporation and did their work correctly, they would receive security, a job for a lifetime, and wage increases that allowed them to have a family.

Think of all the corporations that have merged and the hundreds of thousands of workers that have been fired over the last

25 years. Corporate mergers have caused the displacement of more than 20 million American middle class workers. These people were not emotionally prepared for this. As a result, we are seeing adults as old as forty and fifty moving home with their parents. And their parents are not having an easy time either. In fact, for senior citizens in our society, it is especially difficult. Many elders, who have painstakingly saved all their working lives for their golden years, have seen their retirements wiped out or substantially reduced with their 401K's down about 25%. Who would have thought? The reality is that we can no longer feel really safe, secure, and happy about the prospects of a peaceful and vital future.

Then there is the issue of health. With the passage of time, energetic twenty-somethings, who focus mostly on dating, marriage, family, career advancement, and a better standard of living, become forty- and fifty-year-olds confronted with the more pressing issue of failing health. People who once took their well being for granted now find themselves overweight, fatigued, and suffering from insomnia, mood swings, hot flashes, impotency, arthritis, diabetes, high blood pressure, cancer, and a myriad of other diseases, the result of years of stress, poor lifestyle, and an improper diet.

Americans have difficulty growing older. All things end, but rarely are we prepared for the transitions we must face throughout life and, ultimately, at its end. Frequently once children are grown and gone, parents begin to feel disconnected from a focus that once held meaning and purpose. When we have lost loved ones, either through children leaving the nest, divorce, or death, we don't have a way to properly cope. Nor do we know how to approach the unavoidable conclusion of our own lives, as death is a taboo subject in our youth-oriented society.

Introduction

Millions of seniors are leading lives of quite desperation—sitting at home watching television, the phone seldom ringing, just waiting for the inevitable end at some unknown point in the future. Elders are dealing with a challenge to their emotions. They may feel loneliness and despair in a society that has no value for people who can no longer compete, a separation of their emotional bonds, physical suffering that usually accompanies aging, and a fear of death. Yes, there are those who are still living happily, but they are in the tiny minority compared to those who are costing over one trillion dollars a year in medical expenses. Feeling neglected, sick, and tired, elders may ask, "What is the point of it all anyway?"

There is a pervading atmosphere of despair in our fast-paced world today that was not present in the past even during the hardest of economic times. My parents suffered through the Great Depression and my father went into the Second World War. Despite 16 years of such hardship, they never felt a sense of hopelessness because their optimism and spirit always served as a counterbalance. Plus their money went a long way. My father earned $3,000 a year as a police officer and was able to save enough to provide us with a home, food, and clothing, as did many other fathers and mothers.

In contrast, think of the career woman today: a woman in her thirties with a college degree, family, and career. Imagine the pressure of multi-tasking, of trying to fit everything in some priority of importance in a day's schedule. Think of the stress that is created from trying to get her child into the right preschool, kindergarten, and elementary school, the guilt of not spending quality time with her child, but rather consigning other people to be guardians while she's busy at her workplace. There is little time for the things that make life worthwhile—reading a good book, the special hobby, enjoying cultural events, a quality relationship, quiet down time, candlelit dinners, bubble baths, long walks in the park, a jog on the beach. Nice thoughts, but they are rarely accomplished. More often than not, it's as if a gun goes off, and everyone has to start rushing to get to school or work.

It is rare to find people within the American workforce who say that they are happy with their environment and themselves, who say that they are achieving the things they have wanted to in a way that gives them a quality of life rather than just a standard of living. In today's competitive society, men and women are not allowed to cooperate as much as they are forced to compete. This need to compete challenges people to work harder, to do more, to get ahead and stay ahead, as if all the advantages are somewhere in front of them, and they just haven't worked hard enough to grasp them. And if you have, the moment you stop working, someone else is standing behind you, ready to take it from you. This cycle burns people out.

To dissipate feelings of anxiety some people turn to exercise. Interestingly, when I go to the gym in the early morning, I see a lot of people working out, but they do not have happy faces. What I see is an intensity, as if the people there are burning off stress. When I go to the gym at noon, I see packed yoga classes. But even this is a vigorous, sweat-producing activity. After class, they are rushing back to a toxic and overly stimulating environment. They think of that one hour of yoga as just enough to sublimate the anxiety they are feeling. The gym today is not the environment for socializing that it was in the 1970's. Rather, it's people almost opening a vein on a treadmill to release the toxins of the day.

Their co-workers, on the other hand, may be drinking at a bar to create a buzz that takes the edge off. Or maybe they're smoking marijuana. More Americans are anesthetizing themselves now than ever. And yes, it will take the pain away for a while. But now we know there is paranoia, delusional psychoses, and extreme anxiety or depression caused by its use. When the anxiety or depression comes back after withdrawal from the drug, the only way to get over it is to go back on the drug again, creating perpetual long-term abuse.

Other people will sublimate their anxiety by overeating. They don't really care what their bodies look like and will sit in front of a television set, drink beer, and eat pizza and fried chicken. Women will commensurate with Oprah, Montell, and Dr. Phil, their favorite soap operas and weepy movie where they identify, "Yes, I'm crying with you because my life is something of a reflection." Most men still believe that a real man doesn't cry and show his feelings, and they will displace their feelings by watching sports on television, or working on a car, or going bowling. These are not bad outlets, but rather, one way of taking the edge off of their anxiety and depression.

So, take a look around. See the political and economic instability in the world in which we live, the disintegration of the American family, people working too hard with inadequate support systems. When we look at all the circumstances that are beyond our capacity to manage, we should not wonder why so many Americans feel depressed or anxious.

Another part of the problem in our society, however, is that abnormal life circumstances are viewed as normal situations. We are expected to adjust to them, and if we can't, the fault lies within us, we're told. This way of thinking was prompted several years ago by a massive advertising campaign started by Eli Lilly for Prozac. Lilly tried to make it seem as if depression were the result of a brain chemical imbalance and that by taking their drug we would feel better and resolve the problem. The idea caught on and other conditions were attributed to this inbalance. If a woman had PMS, her brain was imbalanced. If a child asked too many questions, or got up from his seat in the classroom too many times, or asked too many questions, it was because his brain was imbalanced.

Today we've made being a child into a disease and millions of children are labeled with ADD, ADHD, and other fictitious acronyms. In this generation alone we have seven million children on prescription medications each day for the control of their behavior. When I was growing up, you never saw a child being medicated for such a reason. When you had problems, you talked about them to your family over dinner. If there was the need for outside counseling, you generally spoke to your favorite school-teacher or Sunday school teacher, rabbi, or priest. Only if something were really, really bad would you see a psychologist, and that was rarely talked about. It merely happened. Most of the time you were able to understand and work through it, tough it out. Things would get better. Today, nobody asks questions to get to the root of the problem, questions like, "What are you feeding your children?" or "What other drugs are you taking?"

There is enormous evidence supporting the connection between a brain chemistry altered by various substances and a person's mood. Hence, we can artificially create depression or anxiety symptoms by such things as refined sugars, the artificial chemicals added to processed foods, pesticides, milk products, antibiotics, and birth control pills. Ironically, the very drugs purported to help these so-called "ADD" and "ADHD" children may alter brain chemistry and result in depression and anxiety.

Also, you can have medical conditions that have depression or anxiety as a side effect. Often these go undiagnosed. For example, a person goes to a doctor complaining of black moods. The patient is fatigued and overweight and the doctor prescribes an antidepressant when, in fact, it might have been an under active thyroid gland (three symptoms of an under active thyroid gland are depression, fatigue, and overweight). Or the person might be hyperglycemic. Rather than check the blood sugar, the doctor may only look at symptoms and diagnose depression. An antidepressant is prescribed when the cause of the depression, an erratic blood sugar, could have been easily corrected with a simple diet and supplements. What if a child is allergic to milk, and the allergy manifests in the brain and causes hyperactivity? I can assure you that the doctor, psychologist, or school teacher is not going to tell little Jimmy, "Let's check to see if brain allergies are manifesting as a hyperactive reaction to something you have eaten or drank?" No, they're going to say, "Jimmy's ADHD and needs Ritalin." So, our society has taken the cue from the pharmaceutical industry and a compliant medical industry and teaching profession that proports that all of the symptoms of depression and anxiety are real brain abnormalities that need medical attention and drugging. This is unfortunate because it has made us dependent. In effect, it has made us beholding to the psychologists, psychiatrists, primary physicians, pediatricians, and school teachers to tell us what to do, and they all are singing from the same drug handbook.

Of course, nothing changes as the conditions that led to these feelings go unresolved. And frequently we have worse feelings. People, who would have never thought of suicide after taking certain medications, including children, now think of suicide. It's a side effect of psychotropic medications. Children who were not truly depressed frequently become depressed as one of the side effects of antidepressants.

Have these medications been challenged? No. Have any of the true underlying causes of the conditions been looked at? No. Massive PR campaigns back up physicians who prescribe these medications and the pharmaceutical industry who create these drugs and who create the notion that we need them. The National Institute of Mental Health supports them. Nobody wants to take the responsibility for having been wrong. As the legal and political consequences are great, everyone is in denial and nothing gets better.

This book is an extremely honest and meticulous look at what is really causing our troubles, especially the problem of everyone thinking they're depressed or anxious and in need of a medical fix. If I were writing this book 15 years ago, I might have started with a good diet and proper supplementation and ended with exercise and stress management, but today is a different time and requires a different approach, one that truly examines how we have managed in just a 15-year period to virtually pathologize life.

No one is safe from being considered a disease that needs to be treated with appropriate drugs or hospitalization. African Americans, senior citizens, and children have been especially susceptible to the pharmaceutical industry's drugging campaigns. I have therefore written an extended chapter showing how we have abused hundreds of millions of people over the decades without the media, social leaders, even activists being aware of what was happening. If we are to correct the problem we have to face it, and a nutrient is not the only answer.

I then ask and answer a question that has not been asked or answered in any other book that I have read. Is your official medical diagnosis accurate? If not, then the treatment cannot be correct. It has taken me a long time to review the scientific literature to show that across the board, in every single area of medicine, a major fraud has been perpetrated. Therefore, to rely solely on the judgment of your primary care physician could be a fatal mistake. The information here could save you from becoming yet another iatrogenic (medical error) statistic. Think of the millions of American women receiving synthetic hormone replacement therapy who are now shown to have a high incidence of heart disease, cervical cancer and breast cancer because of their medication. I do not want to see any more statistics. Similarly, iatrogenic effects from antidepressants and antipsychotic medications are all too common.

At the other end, I will present scientific literature that supports the use of alternative, natural, nontoxic approaches for dealing with anxiety and depression. We will look at various approaches as we explore guided imagery, neurolinguistic programming, therapeutic touch, tai chi, qi gong, homeopathy, Bach flower remedies, intravenous vitamin drips, detoxification, and supplementation.

Your primary care doctor or psychiatrist will not tell you about SAME, a natural substance that is crucial to virtually every cell in the body. It is a simple combination of the essential amino acid methionine and ATP, which is important as an energy molecule in all living cells. ATP gives needed carbon to certain proteins, fats, RNA and DNA. When SAME donates carbons it keeps transmitters in the brain at an optimal level. It also helps the fat that makes up nerve cell membranes to function in a way that allows the nerves to work properly. Many people walk around with low grades of blue moods. Medicine has given this a name, subsyndromal depression or intermittent recurrent minor depression. This is just a blue mood that 400-500 mg of SAME can effectively overcome. It also works faster than antidepressants without the side effects. (The only person who wouldn't take it is a manic-depressive who is on other medications. You don't want to go off the medications by yourself, as that can be dangerous.)

There is also something as simple as realizing that from Thanksgiving, through Christmas, until springtime, people frequently feel sad. They lose their energy, have difficulty waking in the morning, crave sweets and starches, gain weight, and withdraw from friends. They have a difficult time concentrating or working. Why? SAD, seasonal affective disorder. In the northern states, it's particularly bad, and in Florida and Southern California it's not seen as often. The reason is that a lack of light causes it. To treat SAD, a simple natural protocol of using sunlight can make a big difference, but not if you don't know about it.

We will also discuss the benefits of methylation, the simple transfer of a methyl group, which is one carbon and three hydrogens that travels around the body causing reactions. This transfer is what happens when we detoxify harmful chemicals from the body. Methylation is related to the melatonin and seratonin cycle, and it relates to mood. There are different nutrients in enhanced methylation, like DMG and SAME. There are a variety of studies showing that SAME helps with depression and helps with methylation.

Also, to prove my point that we must approach this problem from a holistic point of view, I will discuss in depth an anti-depression, anti-anxiety study I did with three groups of people. In one group were people given advice on a holistic diet, lifestyle, stress management, behavior modification for dealing with problems in life, plus exercise. In another group, people were just given brain nutrients, ones known to enhance mood, like melatonin, a special form of tryptophane, and co-enzyme Q10. In yet another group, these two approaches were combined and people received both the nutrients and the lifestyle recommendations. In this group, there were tremendous changes. People who had been clinically depressed for 30 years overcame their depression in three months. Clearly, if true brain imbalances were causing depression and anxiety, a lifestyle change would not have made a difference, but it did, proving that these are not brain imbalances but merely ways we can enhance our sense of well being. This is a far better approach for people to take than the current medical model.

In the next chapters of the book I'll present wonderful recipes to bring nutritious, living, cleansing foods back into our diets. In this section, there is great variety from which to choose, and meals that can be made with joy and ease. Whether you are 16 or 60, this should be an important part of the program.

Plus I found that virtually everyone who was depressed or anxious had a defective immune system. Indeed, a side effect of depression is an immune system that plummets, making us more susceptible to diseases of all types. I have therefore included a section on 110 ways to enhance your immunity. Here you will find ways to build your immune system up and keep it strong.

Finally, I have listed positive affirmations. These are my own original affirmations that I have used within my study group. I ask that you take one affirmation per day and focus on it.

In essence, this book is different from others on this subject. It deals with issues that the depressed or anxious person may not have ever thought of before, but it is one that could save your life, or certainly save you from the harm of being misdiagnosed, misprescribed, and mistreated.

* * *

Introduction

Following is an outline of *The Seven Steps to Eliminating Depression and Anxiety Disorders*. Be aware that success in this program requires that a lifestyle modification take place. A lifestyle modification, as the term implies, involves change. And I can't emphasize strongly enough that this change may be uncomfortable, especially if the practices involved are radically new and different from your current way and require frequent daily reminders. In most cases, discomfort should be expected to some degree. If you can get past your "comfort zone" then the results are guaranteed to change your life for the better, but not for good unless you maintain this new approach to life. For example, if you eat hamburgers, hotdogs and barbequed chicken and cannot imagine life without this traditional American cookout fair, then you are most likely in a comfort zone. Remember that if you find it hard to say "no" to something, then you are probably well within your comfort zone and should probably evaluate whether that something could have a negative impact on your life. Think of the changes that are being suggested in this book and if they seem too difficult or uncomfortable and lead to thoughts of delaying the process, then realize the following. The greater your resistance to implementing these steps in your life, the richer and greater the rewards will be in the end. Just as three people who are about to undertake a mountain climbing expedition may each gain different levels of reward from taking the summit and reaching the other side of the mountain, it's the person who had the greatest resistance and desire to climb the mountain that we can objectively say overcame the greatest amount of negativity. And it's this potential of overcoming negativity that is truly valuable in overcoming depression and anxiety disorders. Beyond the purely physical aspects of overcoming this disorder, psychological success, as in achieving a goal, has the potential of releasing regenerative, positive energies that in themselves are pure and healing. And what will the rewards be more specifically? Although they come in many forms, the best possible way to phrase what the outcome of this program is would be to go to the testimonial section of this book. Read about actual changes and the conditions that existed prior to the changes. I'll see you on the other side of the mountain.

Step I: How to Identify and Eliminate Risk Factors—This first step is crucial in determining what foods and other substances might be causing allergic reactions that may very well result in an allergic reaction. Depression or anxiety may be the side effect of an allergic reaction.

One way to identify risk factors is by using the coco pulse test. In the morning upon arising, without getting out of bed, take your pulse. After you take your pulse, place a food that you would like to test for allergic reaction under your tongue. Wait a few minutes. Now take your pulse again. If your pulse increases more than five beats per minute it's quite likely that you are allergic to that food and that food should be eliminated from your diet. Foods that should typically be eliminated or avoided altogether are: animal products, wheat, all dairy, all processed sugars, hydro genated oils, nightshade vegetables and simple carbohydrates like white wheat pasta. Also, note that eating organic foods is very important, since even if you eat a food that is recommended, if that food is loaded with pesticides it will undoubtedly be harmful to you and may cause low grade or even severe allergic reactions.

Step II: Cleansing and Detoxifying—Detoxification involves several systems of the body including the liver, the kidneys, the large intestine, skin, lungs and lymphatic system. Each of these systems can be individually detoxified through various techniques.

Detoxifying the liver, the "workhorse organ," is essential. This can be done through a juice therapy cleanse, whereby you build up to as many vegetable and / or fruit juices you can consume. This cleanse should ideally be scheduled for one week. Meals should be limited to once per day. The balance of your nutrition in this cleanse should come from juices and protein shakes. You can use any quality soy or rice based protein powders. This cleanse should be conducted for one continuous week at least two times per year. Juices may be consumed as frequently as desired.

During this week of detoxification, exercise should be increased in order to enhance the body's cleansing through perspiration and increased circulation. Saunas or hot baths are also suggested in order to detoxify through the skin. Remember not to exceed more than fifteen minutes per sauna session. Always keep well hydrated during heat cleanses. Drink up to one gallon of water or juice per day.

Coffee enemas are also very beneficial for the liver cleanse as well as the large intestine. Organic coffee should be diluted to a light golden color and chilled to room temperature. It can then be administered via an enema, retaining the coffee for a total of fifteen minutes. It may be difficult at first to retain the liquid, so here are a few tips. Do a water enema first, using fresh, clean water at room temperature. This does not have to be retained. It can be released as soon as the urge appears. After the water is fully evacuated, you may administer the coffee, retaining the liquid for five minutes on your right side, five minutes on your back and finally five minutes on you left side. Do not exceed a total of fifteen minutes. Acidophilus and bifidus, the good bacterias, should be consumed after the enema session.

Breathing fully for fifteen minutes daily will help relieve stress as well as re-teach the body to completely exhale carbon dioxide. This will minimize toxic gaseous build-up in the blood, resulting in increased overall energy and greater oxygen utilization.

Following is a kidney cleansing tea that can do wonders. Steep one teaspoon dried dandelion leaf and one teaspoon marshmallow root in a cup of boiling water. Strain, let cool and drink with your preference of a natural sweetener. You may repeat this five times daily. This drink is rich in minerals such as potassium. Herbs have been frequently used in cleansing the kidneys. Dandelion leaf promotes diuresis. Corn silk soothes urinary tract inflammation. The herb bearberry (uva-ursi) has been associated with relieving bladder stone pains and bedwetting.

Red clover is an excellent herb for lymphatic detoxification as well as Echinacea and gingko-biloba.

One of the best ways to help cleanse the lymphatic system is through exercise, especially rebounding and other more high impact routines. If joint problems are a concern, non-impacting exercises such as low-impact aerobics and more vigorous forms of Yoga may be useful as well.

Step III: Rejuvenation—Now that you've cleansed your body internally, its time to incorporate proper nutrients to rejuvenate the integrity of your cells. Remember, it's important to detoxify prior to beginning a nutritional protocol because most of the nutrients that you consume will be assimilated in the large intestine. Please review the anxiety and depression protocols recommended later in this book. Begin taking the supplements one at a time, building the recommended dosages slowly as well.

Step IV: De-Stressing Our Lives—The number one killer disease in the United States is not cancer, heart disease, AIDS or any other disease that is commonly in the social consciousness. The number one killer disease is stress, which exacerbates most maladies and reduces the immune system, making the body susceptible to the occurrence of factors that contribute to an array of other conditions. This is why the mother of all diseases can most certainly be called "stress."

So what can a person do to control this killer? First of all, it's important to note that stress in and of its self can be useful. It's ultimately the way stressful circumstances are perceived in ones life that can make a difference. For example, consider two people who have to give a public speech. One individual is confident and enjoys speaking while the other is more reserved, shy and fearful of saying the wrong thing. They both have the same task at hand, yet the individual that is fearful will produce cortisol, a biochemical associated with the development of heart disease. Recurrences of similarly stressful situations in that person's life could ultimately lead to the development of depression as well.

There are many approaches that can be taken in reducing negative reactions to stressful situations. One, for example is prayer. Many studies have been conducted on the power of prayer. You need not be religious in order to speak to a higher power. Just acknowledging that there is a higher power which may guide ones life could be a relief in and of itself. Letting go of the ego and allowing your image of a higher power show you the next obstacle, hurdle or challenge is a refreshing viewpoint to begin with. Then asking that higher power for guidance with absolute faith that you are being listened to can displace your dependence from wanting to always be in control. Only then will it be possible to innately listen for direction.

Other methods of stress management are meditation, Qi-gong, Tai-Chi, Yoga, laughter, herbs such as valerian, skull cap herb, St.

John's Wort, Lemon Balm, chamomile and nutrients such as GABA and threonine are very useful too. I can't emphasize strongly enough that you must choose some form of stress management on a regular basis and stick with it. The more you practice, the better you feel and releasing stress will become second nature. I've created a series of videos and audio tapes that address self-empowerment and stress management issues these are helpful tools to introduce fresh perspectives on how to manage stress by shifting your entire paradigm so that you can recognize yourself and your true roles in all that you can touch in your life while maintaining a compassionate heart for all.

Step V: Removing Toxins from Personal and Home Environment—Go through your home and take inventory of all potential environmental toxins. Toxins could be found in places you don't even expect. Dust and mold has to be reduced or eliminated by themselves because they can could cause severe immune responses resulting in disease. You must replace chemical-laden toothpastes, cosmetics, and mouthwashes with natural products. Eliminate the use of fluoride. Shop for organic whole foods. Even the garments you wear should be considered. It's best to wear or use as bedding, cotton, silk and other natural fibers. These fibers should ideally be untreated by chemicals. Buy a quality air and water purification unit. Never drink tap water. These are just a few recommendations. Outline the variables that compose your environment and research the constituents. This approach will prepare you to always question environmental surroundings and avoid personal environmental toxicity for life.

Step VI: Exercise—It is common knowledge these days that exercise is important for optimal health. But what kind of exercise and how frequently should it be done? When considering exercise, we must consider movements that benefit our cardiovascular system and lymphatic system as well as overall muscular strength and endurance. Aerobic exercise in all of it's forms will typically address cardiovascular improvements as well as lymphatic stimulation.

- Though the choices of aerobic exercise may vary greatly, and include activities as running, power walking, swimming, bicycling, cross-country skiing, floor aerobics, Tae Bo, using aerobic machines such as stair masters or versa climbers, and the list goes on, the formula for ensuring that your aerobic work is optimally effective is as follows. Aerobic exercise should begin at 10-20 minutes five days a week and built up to approximately 45–60 minutes five days a week.
- Keeping your heart rate in an aerobic zone is the key to proper aerobic training. The aerobic zone is the optimal beats your heart makes per minute, sustained over the course of your workout. For example, your resting heart rate might be seventy beats per minute but during your work out, the heart rate should increase to a suitable level for your age.
- To find your target heart rate, subtract your age from the number 220, this will give you your maximal heart rate. Now calculate 75% of your maximal heart rate and that result will be your average target heart rate. For senior citizens or individuals who are overweight by at least twenty pounds, the percentage that should be calculated is 65%. Athletes can calculate 85–90%. For example, a senior citizen who is 70 years old would calculate the following: $220 - 70 = 150$, $150 \times 65\% = 97.5$, or rounded up to 98 beats per minute. Now if the senior citizen being discussed is in good shape, he or she

may calculate 75% of the maximal heart rate. So this senior citizen should exercise aerobically for 45–60 minutes maintaining a heart rate of 98 beats per minute for the majority of the work out. This would be a healthy aerobic work out.

Strength training is also important. Again, there are a variety of exercises to choose from calisthenics to Pilates but probably the most effective and easily applicable technique is weight training. There are many good books and videos on weight training that would go into more detail than I wish to dedicate in this book. So do your research and if there's one important tip that I can give about weight training, is that whatever you do, maintain proper posture and fluid breathing in whatever exercise you choose. And even though you must work at a good intensity, enough to eventually break you into a sweat, always remember: Train—Don't Strain!

Step VII: No More Excuses—As I mentioned earlier in this chapter, reaching beyond your "comfort zone" is probably the single most important concept that needs to be understood and applied in order to maintain the lifestyle modifications that I am suggesting. Everyday, all that we do is just a series of choices. We have the ability to choose what is good and positive in every moment. If this is so, then why don't we always choose what is good and positive but instead frequently settle on choices that are ultimately self-destructive? This is the "comfort zone" that I am referring to.

It is quite possible that because of your conditioning, which typically comes from your upbringing and other similar factors, your "comfortable" choices, the ones that you've been accustomed to, are not quite the best ones for your optimal health, friendships, love relationships and even your finances. Identifying where you have a certain "rub" or "discomfort" is step one in releasing yourself from the cycle that you are in. Remember: The mind that caused the problem can never be the mind that solves the problem. So in order to switch from the mind that created the problem to one that can solve it undoubtedly requires a sensation of "discomfort."

The very first thought and place to begin is "No More Excuses." What this means is that you must begin to aggressively and ruthlessly seek out all conditions and cycles in your life that don't contribute to your optimal well being and the joy and sharing that you can experience among other people. Don't allow an excuse to get in your way in starting on the right track, such as; I don't have enough money or I don't have enough time or I'll start next week (which usually means never) or I can't do it alone, and the list can go on as long as there are excuses. But what if you didn't allow for any excuses? What if that was a possibility? Well then guess what—you WILL succeed at this program AND any other task you wish to undertake in your life. It's so easy and comfortable to procrastinate, so reach out, without any excuses, for the great potential that you innately have.

1

RE-EXAMINING THE TRUE NATURE
OF DEPRESSION AND ANXIETY

THERE is an incredible increase in the number of people who are suffering from anxiety and depression. Instead of studying the reasons for this increase society seems to think they have the answer to the problem of anxiety and depression in the form of a pill. But what can we learn from studying the history of depression? There was a time when depression was categorized as mental illness causing the patient to be shunned from society. Even into the 1970s people would never admit to seeing a psychiatrist or taking anti-depressant medication. We used to have human services where real people counseled face-to-face others who had psychological imbalance. Part of the rise in the field of psychiatry itself may stem from people having less personal interaction with older, wiser relatives and friends. When our days are so congested with the responsibilities of work and family, we barely have time to talk to our own partner or children. We hire psychiatrists to perform the service of a kindly aunt or uncle. But they are letting us down and spend less and less time in talk therapy. And with the advent of psychiatric medication for anxiety and depression the talk therapy was put aside and drug therapy became the key to treatment. Mental illness was defined as either a brain disorder or a chemical imbalance with the end result of applying a drug to a particular diagnosis.

Whereas infectious diseases are said to be the result of an external germ invading the physical body, mental illness is thought to be something that develops from a problem within the brain or within the brain chemistry. This is an interesting twist on the mind-body separation in allopathic medicine. The physical body is attacked from without but the mind is attacked from within. Of course, this is true when the outside world can trigger a stress reaction and set the stage for anxiety or depression.

Once it was found that serotonin was a mood-elevating brain neurotransmitter, serotonin deficiency became the diagnosis of chemical imbalance that could cause depression. Because of the mind-body split it was not thought possible that a bad diet, nutrient deficiency, or exposure to noxious chemicals could affect the mind. The cause of the chemical imbalance in the brain was not investigated. What was important was that there was a chemical imbalance in the brain that could possibly be treated by drugs that would eliminate that imbalance. Scientists set out specifically to create such a drug and succeeded with the invention of Prozac.

Even though depression is said to be a chemical imbalance, the diagnosis does not involve measuring the brain chemistry. It's just taken for granted that serotonin deficiency causes depression. So, if a person presents with symptoms that resemble depression, they are depressed, and are given anti-depressant medications. All the while, a mind-boggling number of causes of those symptoms of depression could be occurring but doctors are frequently missing the real cause when they primarily treat the symptoms.

The Diagnostic and Statistical Manual of Mental Disorders, fourth edition (DSM-IV) contains the diagnostic criteria for anxiety and depression. The list is expanding all the time. Recently Premenstrual Syndrome (PMS) was elevated to the status of mental illness. And just in time because once you have the disease you can offer the treatment. Serafem is Prozac disguised as a new treatment for PMS.

The patent for Prozac is running out and a new diagnostic indication for a drug, in this case PMS, means that the patent can be extended on the new drug. Most women know when their period is coming with a little aching in the low abdomen or leg muscles, some mood change, and a feeling like they need to slow down and relax a bit. But that's not always possible in our overly-commercialized and sped-up society. We're conditioned to think we can't slow down for a minute and if we do then we'll miss out on being responsible.

We are pulled along in the rat race to the point where we don't have time to go through normal life processes or have time to process our own feelings. Menopause and PMS are both considered diseases today and each have their medical treatments so they won't "interfere" with our lives. But we forget that our lives are about feelings and interaction and communication. If we don't have time for these normal events and just take medications to suppress feelings, we are living on a very superficial plane of existence.

Children, unfortunately, have been drawn into the drug business as well. Outside school they spend their time watching TV, on the Internet, and playing video games. They also drink a lot of soda with sugar or aspartame sweetener, eat hot dogs dyed with food coloring, eat enormous amounts of bread and pastry ending up with vitamin and mineral deficiencies, all of which affect their mental functioning. Inside school their brains are no longer stimulated in the same way by electronic, digital, and dietary input and they get antsy. Or they cycle with extreme highs and lows. Alert to "abnormal" behavior the teacher and school nurse regularly single out kids who can't pay attention, disrupt the class, or demand attention to the school psychologist. Usually "problem kids" are put on Ritalin under the guise of wanting them to focus on their schoolwork. But no studies have even shown that Ritalin improves a child's learning. It just calms them down enough that they no longer disrupt the class or the teacher's set way of teaching.

Once a child grows up on Ritalin, it's not a huge leap for them to accept antidepressants in their young adult life. They have grown up on drugs and if they find they can't cope with the normal stresses and strains of daily living they fall easily into the habit of taking a mood-elevating drug.

Twenty-five years ago major clinical medical texts listed several types of depression: depressive neurosis, reactive depression, involutional melancholia, manic depressive psychosis, and major affective disorder psychosis. Outside the depressive category altogether was a condition called transient situational disturbances. Depressive neurosis was said to be an hysterical reaction to a transient situational disturbance such as death in the family or other major episode of grief. Reactive depression was also related to reaction to grief. Involutional melancholia was the term used for depression, which occurred around menopause. Major affective disorder psychosis was the name given to depression occurring for no known cause.

Presently depression is categorized as major depression, dysthymia, and bipolar. According to the NIH, major depression is diagnosed when a person has many of the following list of symptoms interfering with the ability to work, study, sleep, eat, and enjoy life:

a. Persistent sad, anxious, or "empty" mood
b. Feelings of hopelessness, pessimism
c. Feelings of guilt, worthlessness, helplessness

   d. Loss of interest or pleasure in hobbies and activities that were once enjoyed, including sex
   e. Decreased energy, fatigue, being "slowed down"
   f. Difficulty concentrating, remembering, making decisions
   g. Insomnia, early-morning awakening, or oversleeping
   h. Appetite and/or weight loss or overeating and weight gain
   i. Thoughts of death or suicide; suicide attempts
   j. Restlessness, irritability
   k. Persistent physical symptoms that do not respond to treatment, such as headaches, digestive disorders, and chronic pain

Dysthymia is a term that wasn't even in use twenty-five years ago and greatly widens the definition of depression. It is said to be a less severe type of depression that involves long-term, chronic symptoms. These symptoms are not disabling but keep a person from functioning well or from "feeling good." Dysthymia as defined in the American Psychiatric Association and International Classification of Mental Disorders as "a prevalent form of subthreshold depressive pathology with gloominess, anhedonia, low drive and energy, low self-esteem and pessimistic outlook."

Bipolar disorder is another name for manic depression and defines mood cycles from manic highs to depressive lows. Bipolar is the least common of the three types of depression occurring in 1.2 % of the population. Major depression occurs in 5% and dysthymia in .4%. In manic depressives. when depressed, the symptoms of depression manifest, when manic the following symptoms are found:

   a. Abnormal or excessive elation
   b. Unusual irritability
   c. Decreased need for sleep

d. Grandiose notions
e. Increased talking
f. Racing thoughts
g. Increased sexual desire
h. Markedly increased energy
i. Poor judgment
j. Inappropriate social behavior

Mania, however, is not the same as anxiety. While depression affects over 40 million American adults, anxiety disorders affect half as many. The anxiety disorders discussed include: panic disorder, obsessive-compulsive disorder, post-traumatic stress disorder, social phobia (or social anxiety disorder), specific phobias, and generalized anxiety disorder (GAD). People with anxiety disorders demonstrate excessive, irrational fear and dread.

The use of drug therapy for anxiety and depression, on the surface, actually suits both patient and doctor. Doctors like it because they think they see fast relief of their patients' symptoms and they can process more needy patients. Previously talk therapy might take several hours a week to perform but once the initial diagnosis was made and a patient put on anti-depressant pills, they would only have to be seen for a few minutes a month or even every three months to renew their prescriptions. Some patients love it because they never have to address the reasons why they're depressed. They imagine they have a chemistry imbalance and are treating it with the proper chemical. Also, patients often can't afford talk therapy. Talking to a psychiatrist for one or two hours a week can be very expensive compared to a prescription-renewal appointment.

Frequently, anxiety and depression have become diagnoses but really they are a psychological reaction. You may be reacting to losing your job, or the death of a family member, or having a fight with your partner or children. And yes, this may make you feel down in the dumps, but it doesn't mean you're clinically depressed. You may even say, "I'm depressed," but it's just a term you use to get the point across instead of going into the details.

When psychiatrists define depression they use the Diagnostic and Statistical Manual of Mental Disorders, fourth edition (DSM-IV). They are very serious about diagnosing depression and categorizing your symptoms because once you are in a particular box your diagnosis can be matched with an "appropriate" drug. So, perhaps we are talking about two types of depression, which are becoming interchangeable. The ups and downs of everyday existence are being swept into the psychiatric definition of severe depression.

Along with the ups and downs of everyday existence are the ups and downs of normal neurotransmitters and natural chemicals in the body. In the 1980s depression was equated with a deficiency of the neurotransmitter, serotonin, in the body. Immediately pharmaceutical companies sought a drug that would elevate serotonin levels. What they didn't do was try to find the reasons why. They didn't look at normal body chemistry; they didn't investigate the vitamins, minerals, amino acids, and essential fatty acids—the nutrients responsible for creating serotonin in the first place.

When you look at anxiety and depression from a whole-body perspective you see that it can be triggered in dozens of ways. Chemical imbalance at the neurotransmitter can be caused by too much sugar in the diet, wheat/gluten allergy, mold allergy, excess alcohol intake, vitamin deficiency, mineral deficiency, essential fatty acid deficiency, amino acid deficiency, chemical allergies (additives and colorings), exposure to toxic chemicals and heavy metals, side effects of almost any prescription medication. But when the sole treatment for chemical imbalance is thought to be synthetic drugs, we lose sight of the delicate biochemistry of the mind and body that can be manipulated by food and other medications.

How can a drug possibly help you get over being worried about financial insecurity? When you have such a problem you want to be sharp as a tack to solve it. Instead you are put on a medication that creates an emotional detachment from your problems; you just don't care anymore.

What are we to make of a recent study, which showed that a placebo was even more effective in helping people with depression than Prozac? There are several aspects to consider. It certainly makes you wonder whether the drug is doing anything at all. If the placebo works better, then the drug was actually making people feel worse. Also the study showed that there were brain chemistry changes attributable to the placebo that were identical to changes with the drug. But what they are forgetting is that anyone who takes any pill, whether placebo or medication, is going to have a placebo effect.

The placebo effect occurs when a person's own healing mechanisms are triggered. Thinking you are taking a pill that will help you stimulates you to help yourself. Modern medicine has forgotten that the most important aspect of treating patients is to develop a rapport and let the patient know you want to help them. With the rise of HMO's and the mechanization of medicine doctors are only given minutes to spend with a patient and increasingly have become prescription drug prescribers. They no longer have quality time to spend getting to know their patients. Knowing about someone's job, their family, their diet, and their goals are very important ways of connecting with a patient and also help a doctor make the right diagnosis.

If your doctor knows that you work in a toxic environment, that can help him or her decide whether you are suffering irritability and depression due to toxic chemicals. Knowing that you drink 10 cups of coffee a day can certainly help your doctor decide that's what may be triggering your heart palpitations and feelings of anxiety. Knowing your father just died after a lengthy illness can help your doctor decide that you're going through a normal grieving process superimposed on exhaustion for which you need time off from work, not a drug prescription.

Family-oriented "Marcus Welby" medicine seems beyond our reach now. Instead television drug ads make the diagnosis of anything from PMS to heartburn and gastrointestinal problems, to anxiety and depression right on the screen. Drug companies know that people spend most of their free time sitting in front of the television. They also know that television puts people in a receptive and suggestible mode. The entertainment content of television also plays a part. The dramas are often violent and depressing and the sitcoms are sugar-coated mini-dramas where all the problems in the family are worked over in a half hour. After a while you become conditioned to think that you too are depressed and that there are easy solutions to your problems. Those solutions are the ads. It would be interesting to do a study to see where TV ads for antidepressants are placed. Are they more predominant in sitcoms or in dramas? Are they placed nearer the end of dramas when people feel more burdened with the weight of the problems on the screen and need a quick-fix solution?

When television ads give a list of anxiety or depression symptoms, most people automatically identify with those symptoms. Especially when those symptoms are so generalized that they fit the majority of our population. "Are you feeling stressed? Are you losing sleep due to worrying? Do you want help?" YES, YES, YES. These ads, according to the drug companies are having the desired effect of people marching into their doctor's offices demanding medications to make them feel good. And they might feel good initially. Perhaps it's due to the placebo effect, and perhaps because they weren't depressed in the first place. But they think someone listened to them, even for only a short time, and a doctor gave them something to make them feel better.

The placebo effect kicks in and they perk up, for a time. But then, echoing in the background is the rapid-fire list of side effects that the drug companies are required to recite during their commercial. It goes something like: this drug can cause nausea, vomiting, diarrhea, constipation, anaphalactic shock, and symptoms up to and including death. In men it's impotence, which is a big shock. If he keeps taking the drug after the disfuntion only because he happened to be in for a prescription renewal and told his doctor who had the immediate answer to his problem. Viagra was the answer.

Now, he was already taking tums and metamucil for the drying effects of the medication that made him feel nauseous and gave him constipation. But what he didn't know was that the calcium carbonate in the antiacid tablet was neutralizing his stomach acid and he wasn't digesting his food properly. Gradually he became more fatigued and lethargic because he wasn't absorbing nutrients from his undigested food. In order to cope with that he drank more coffee and ate more sweets. Then he knew he was really depressed and anxious as well because he began to gain weight and now had heart palpitations. Never once did he realize these symptoms were all a result of the antiacid tablet. Or that he was developing hypoglycemia from the excessive sugar in his diet. Or that he was deficient in magnesium, which can cause heart symptoms. Neither did his doctor know what was really going on; he or she never asked him about their patient's diet but instead prescribed heart medications for the palpitations and an anxiolytic drug for the anxiety.

Viagra in a patient with heart symptoms is a possible contraindication but the doctor had forgotten he had given his patient a renewable prescription. Each drug that was added was justified in the doctor's chart and by the HMO billing codes. Each drug was adding to the patient's toxicity and putting increasing strain on the liver's capacity to detoxify.

When drug companies list side effects in the Physician's Desk Reference (PDR) they happily do so because if the side effect is listed, then it's difficult to prevail if you sue. They have reported the side effect and the doctor at least should be aware of what's been reported. But the doctor doesn't necessarily read about every drug he prescribes, and most patients have no idea that they could be taking a "time bomb." Even if they are aware of side effects some patients feel it won't happen to them and some have been made complacent by the amount of drugs in use today. Patients often feel that if a drug is prescribed by a doctor it must be safe. They don't realize that almost half of the drugs that reach the market are removed or relabeled within 10 years for dangerous side effects. In the intervening ten years the number of fatalities and adverse reactions add up.

In the field of nutritional medicine with its common knowledge of dozens of alternatives to drugs, it's hard to imagine how a person can rationalize taking drugs with even a glimmer of side effects much less drugs that, by verified reports, cause over 100,000 deaths and 2 million severe reactions annually. What are people thinking? Well, perhaps they're thinking that someone else is doing the thinking for them. Maybe they're thinking that medicine has their best interests in mind and that doctors are there to help them. They've grown up on Marcus Welby, Dr. Kildare, and ER and think doctors are heroes. It's the Baby Boomer generation that has grown up on wild expectations of a great life. Growing up on drugs the boomers learned to medicate each stage of life, and now they have the expectation that they would be taken care of in their old age with free medications. Boomers, busy following their "bliss", allowed their children and grandchildren be put on Ritalin and now Prozac. They resent the Generation Xers and their dotcom millions and try to stay on top of their game with Prozac and Viagra.

Doctors in the meanwhile have become disenfranchised from their Marcus Welby roots. They've become employees of HMO's unable to make even the simplest of decisions regarding the welfare of their patients. Most doctors have no awareness of the mind-body connection or that food, chemicals, and drugs can cause depression. But in the current HMO settings with appointment times running about seven minutes, there is not even time for a friendly interaction with patients that might be reassuring to patients undergoing stress. Now they are faced with doctors who are as stressed as they are.

In this book we point out that depression is being vastly over diagnosed, vastly overmedicated, and alternative therapies are being completely ignored by mainstream medicine. But it gets worse. Even if a doctor knows that anxiety and depression can be caused by hypoglycemia, nutrient deficiencies, or chemical intoxication, he or she may not be allowed to do the appropriate testing to make the proper diagnosis. An HMO clerk can unilaterally make a decision that a particular request for a glucose tolerance test for an anxious or depressed patient doesn't fall into the criteria of tests that can be ordered for anxiety or depression. He or she cancels the test. Otherwise the patient has to pay out of pocket. If a doctor orders vitamin and mineral blood tests for a depressed patient and the HMO clerk doesn't find those tests on the "approved" list the same thing happens–the test is cancelled. If a doctor orders blood tests for heavy metals, thinking that mercury or lead toxicity could play a role in his patient's depression the test will likely be cancelled.

As long as the prevailing opinion in the medical community is that depression is caused by a serotonin deficiency, and even though serotonin is rarely tested in the patient, then any other tests are deemed unnecessary. If a doctor tries to fight for these tests for his patients he usually wastes his time or even worse, his behavior sets off a red-flag warning at HMO headquarters. Similarly, if a doctor writes letters on a patient's behalf to recover money spent on tests not covered by the patient's insurance, the doctor's billing practices are carefully scrutinized. If the doctor falls outside the "standard practice of medicine" by ordering unapproved tests, using unapproved treatments, or even by not prescribing as many drugs as his peers, he can be brought before his state medical board to answer such charges. Health care should largely be the responsibility of the individual, but when doctors are routinely disciplined when they try to avoid giving drugs to their patients it makes it impossible for patients to find a doctor sympathetic to alternatives. And it means that doctors are never going to be able to make any changes in the system. They are too vulnerable to their medical board, they can lose their license and their livelihood too easily for sticking their necks out.

So, it's up to you, readers. It's up to you to understand the problem we are facing in our health care system. It's up to you to take a stand, to take charge of your health and your health care. To give you ammunition and support for your own healing this book reviews hundreds of studies proving the effectiveness and safety of alternative therapies for anxiety and depression. Start with the basics, a good organic diet, natural supplements, exercise, and simple relaxation techniques and you'll be amazed at how much better you feel.

2

THE PROBLEM WITH
THE DIAGNOSIS

THE Washington Post ran a series of articles on depression from January to May 2002. In his January 9th article staff writer Shankar Vedantam reports on a study showing a three-fold increase in drug therapy for depression from 1987 to 1997. Vedantam feels that, "The sea change probably does not stem from an actual increase in depression." And he makes an impressive list of the possible causes for this unprecedented rise in medical intervention into the moods and emotions of our population. He says, "Instead, it is most likely connected to the destigmatization of mental health problems in general and depression in particular, the rise of managed-care insurance plans, and the arrival of powerful drugs including Prozac, accompanied by multimillion-dollar marketing campaigns." [1]

It is true that managed care has effectively systematized mental health care into a primarily drug-based treatment approach, which is much cheaper than extended psychotherapy or hospitalization. Mr. Vedantam reports that about one third of patients in 1987 were prescribed medications whereas in 1997 three-quarters were prescribed medications and saw their doctor only two thirds of the time of the 1987 patients. Treatment also shifted from psychiatrists to primary care physicians and other health care providers. Vedantam said there was concern by psychiatrists that some of the patients may not be getting the treatment they need, and that some might be getting misdiagnosed or over-diagnosed by unqualified people. The psychiatrists, who do more psychotherapy than general practitioners, are concerned not just about patients being mistreated but also about losing their incomes.

In a May 21st *Washington Post* article Shankar Vedantam again tackles the topic of depression.[2] He says that about 19 million people suffer from depression and almost two-thirds receive no treatment. Depression is being called the most common and the most untreated chronic disease. But help is on the way, mostly in the form of drug therapy, from "a top independent advisory panel" who recommend that doctors begin routinely screening all patients for depression, saying that: "America's primary care doctors are missing and mistreating more than half of all cases of the common mental disorder."

This panel is the government-funded U.S. Preventive Services Task Force, a "highly influential group of scientists that sets widely followed standards on topics ranging from prostate cancer screenings to mammograms." Presumably the panel is not funded by the drug-industry, but investigating their mandate we find that they are all university-based and hospital-based medical doctors. Most university and hospital research is primarily funded by drug companies. So, from all appearances this panel is going to do nothing more than promote drug-therapy for depression. Where are the Naturopaths who detoxify and supplement depressed patients, the Clinical Ecologists who examine brain allergies as a cause of depression, the Certified Clinical Nutritionists who look at nutritional aspects of depression? When all you have is a hammer, everything looks like a nail. Allopathic medicine has elevated drugs to the status of hammer against the nail of depression.

What's really of concern is the way this task force hopes to swell the ranks of depressed people being treated. They say that every patient should be asked two basic questions on every visit to determine whether they are depressed:

1. "Over the past two weeks, have you felt down, depressed or hopeless?"
2. "Over the past two weeks, have you felt little interest or pleasure in doing things?"

The task force advises that if the problems have lasted throughout the previous two weeks, and have interfered with the patient's ability to perform day-to-day tasks, doctors may make a diagnosis of depression.

Who hasn't had a time when they felt down, or little pleasure in doing things? Does that mean we are all depressed? Maybe that's just the point, maybe we are all supposed to be on Prozac—from a marketing point of view!

What other factors in our environment and culture make us depressed and subject to drug intervention. Let's look at our major forms of cultural entertainment, movies and television. For example, Woody Allen and his characterization of "modern man" greatly helped with the destigmatization of mental health problems making everyone feel less neurotic and depressed than he or his characters. He made a visit to the psychiatrist a "normal" event. In the movie *Shampoo*, someone during a panic attack cried out, "has anyone got a Valium" followed by a showering of prescription bottles. Now Prozac is the drug de jour. Antianxiety and antidepressant drugs are part of the cultural norm.

Ann Landers, in her popular advice column in 1998, maintained that "80 percent of people with depression can be treated successfully with medication, psychotherapy or a combination of

The Problem with the Diagnosis

the two."[3] In that year she reported there were 17 million depressed Americans. She was an enthusiastic proponent of medical intervention for depression when she reported that on National Depression Screening Day in 1997, more than 85,000 people visited screening sites. She said that for the 1998 National Depression Screening Day on October 8 there would be more than 3,000 free anonymous screening sites all across the country that everyone should attend.

National Depression Screening Day was originated by the US Dept of Health and Human Services National Institute of Mental Health, which is now only one of the many sponsors of the program. The program is run by Screening for Mental Health, Inc. (SMH) (formerly the National Mental Illness Screening Project), "a nonprofit organization developed to coordinate nationwide mental health screening programs and to ensure cooperation, professionalism, and accountability in mental illness screenings." SMH also claims to be involved in several research initiatives that are shedding new light on America's mental health. SMH admits that their programs are supported solely through grants, donations, and registration fees from participating screening sites. Some of their sponsors include: Eli Lilly, Pfizer, Abbott Laboratories, Solvay Pharmaceuticals, Forest Laboratories, GlaxoSmithKline, Organon Increase, and Wyeth Pharmaceuticals. [4]

Eli Lilly makes Prozac—for depression, obsessive-compulsive disorder (OCD), bulimia (including long-term treatment) and panic disorder; Sarafem—for premenstrual dysphoric disorder (PMDD); and Zyprexa—for schizophrenia and acute bipolar mania. Pfizer makes Zoloft and Viagra. These companies provide the educational material and funding for over 5,000 depression testing sites for National Depression Screening Day. A new initiative has installed 500 high schools with depression testing sites.

In 2001 the National Depression Screening Day was mounted "to educate the public about depression and its symptoms and to encourage individuals to be screened." However, their goals in 2002 were much loftier. They described National Depression Screening Day as "an effort to educate the public nationwide about depression, bipolar disorder (also called manic-depression), anxiety, and post-traumatic stress disorder." [5]

Such screening days under the guise of helping the public deal with symptoms of depression may be more about drug companies having access to millions of consumers who may be gullible enough to think that life can be enhanced with a pill.

Yes, the major destigmatization of mental health has come from pharmaceutical companies who, according to Mr. Vedantam, offer powerful drugs including Prozac and promote them by multimillion-dollar marketing campaigns, especially on the powerful medium of television. As people sit in front of the TV screen, appearing like couch potatoes, they already have a drug surging in their brains. It's called dopamine.[6] Dopamine creates feelings of alertness, excitement, and aggression. When separated from their TV-drug fix, and not knowing they are coming down from a TV-high, people feel depressed and feel they need a drug. They reach for carbohydrates, which increase the levels of serotonin in their brains, and they fill prescriptions for Prozac to revive that "feel-good" sense.

What did people do in times of great stress in the past? In the great wars, in the great depression, were people tougher then? Have the privileges of the baby-boomer generation somehow weakened the resolve needed to cope with everyday stresses and everyday emotions without caving in?

Through the years the increase in anxiety and depression has been blamed on stress. But the obvious fact that we consume more information than previous generations has often been cited as causing stress. We see a horror movie and think we've lived it, our adrenal glands get hammered by the images, adrenaline shoots through our body and speeds up our heart. When it's all over we feel let down. Every time we see a thrilling event on television we go through the same roller coaster, but we have no idea how it's affecting our body chemistry. If it is a horrible world event that we witness, we go through our personal emotions, but then because the media uses these disasters for content to sell advertising, we relive and rehash these events over and over until we are exhausted, both physically and mentally. When Lady Diana died and with the September 11th tragedy, armies of reporters and psychiatrists tried to tell us how we were feeling and bathed our raw nerves with more information than we could handle. When you go through an event and it is replayed into your brain a thousand times, we could assume it has a deep impact on your psyche.

There's more afoot than just being brainwashed by TV. Why are people watching so much TV in the first place? Are we a nation where people have just too much time on their hands? The content of a normal brain is worry. But if we busy ourselves with our job, families, and the daily crises that occur we don't pay much attention to the incessant nagging. The baby boomers with their life-long desires—not to work as hard as their parents, not to be involved with a war, not to work all their lives in a dead-end job that they hate, not to go through another Great Depression—have in fact evoked the opposite. They have created personal depression on a massive scale. They are not content with their lives. And the pharmaceutical companies have marketed this discontent and made them feel that the symptoms can be alleviated by drugs—a mantra reminding us of Soma, the drug given to pacify the population in Orwells' book *1984*.

3

PATHOLOGIZING LIFE

THERE is a crisis in the United States today. Forty million of its citizens are diagnosed as having depression. An increasing number of these are children, the elderly, and African-Americans. But this statistic occurs in a society that in the past decade has witnessed unparalleled growth in the wealth of services, information, and consumer choices, especially in the realm of health One just has to think of the number of pharmacies that have sprung up in your neighborhood, whether it's in a large city or small town. One would suppose that our health is being properly serviced. So why are we losing the battle for people's general well being as shown by recent data?

Looking back, the United States experienced many depressing events in the past century: the Depression, two world wars, and many smaller wars that directly affected the well being and mental health of its citizenry. But somehow they were able to cope without being labeled "ill". They may have experienced many painful emotions, but these didn't require medications or therapies, in general. Today, in a time of unprecedented prosperity, however, more and more people are being classified as incapable of coping with their daily routines and circumstances, and, therefore, requiring treatment, usually in the form of pharmaceuticals.

Now into this contemporary situation is dropped an informational bomb. On June 13, 2002, ABC News.com announced that recent studies show that placebos (sugar pills) can often be just as effective at improving mood, and even brain chemistry, as some of the most widely advertised and prescribed drugs in the country. The report stressed that placebos have been underestimated as a form of treatment for depression. But we think the more relevant insight gleaned from these results is that the patients aren't really sick, ill, or "depressed" in the first place. These studies, if interpreted in this light, then reveal a very disturbing pattern: we are pathologizing life. In this section we will show, by examining trends in medication for children, African-Americans, and the elderly, that our claim is not hysterical, but it is the professional functionaries in sociology, psychology, psychiatry, and medicine that can be accused of overreacting and consequently over prescribing for normal moods, feelings, and sensations—in other words, the average spectrum of reactions to being alive.

For example, as we navigate our way into the 21st century, there is an ominous trend that, strangely, doesn't seem to concern people as much as it should: Millions of children are now taking psychotropic drugs. And they're not doing it illegally, but by prescription. In fact, the medical and educational establishments are conducting a skyrocketing campaign to get kids, and their parents, to "just say yes" to brain-altering pharmaceuticals, with the drug of choice being Ritalin. In 1970, when approximately 150,000 students were on Ritalin, America was alarmed enough to get the Drug Enforcement Agency to classify Ritalin and other amphetamine-type drugs as Class II substances, a category that includes cocaine and one that indicates significant risk of abuse. Despite this apparent safeguard, the number of children taking psychiatric stimulants today has risen over 40-fold; current estimates are that between 6 and 7 million children are taking them.[1]

The American Academy of Pediatrics estimates that as many as 3.8 million school children, mostly boys, are currently diagnosed with attention deficit hyperactivity disorder, and that at least a million children take Ritalin, a figure that many regard as a gross underestimate. And it is not just schoolchildren who are being dosed with psychotropics: Even preschoolers—those aged 2 to 4—experienced a tripling of such prescriptions in a recent five-year period.[2]

Exactly why is all this juvenile pill-popping a problem? Well, for one thing, Ritalin is a drug that has a more potent effect on the brain than cocaine.[3] And we're supposed to be a country that eschews the use of such mind-altering substances, certainly for children. For another, Ritalin's side effects can range from unwelcome personality changes to cardiovascular problems to death. Plus there's the very real issue of whether the "diseases" for which this powerful medicine is prescribed are in fact real diseases at all.

The problem becomes further complicated when you consider that, in addition to the Ritalin explosion, increasing numbers of children are also being prescribed antidepressants, and that these are drugs originally designed and tested for adults. (A fact not generally publicized is that it's legal to prescribe drugs "off label," that is, for conditions or populations that they weren't originally designed for.) So in 1996, over 700,000 children and adolescents were taking Prozac and similar antidepressants in the SSRI group, an 80-percent increase from just two years earlier. It's not that the SSRI's have been proven effective in battling childhood and adolescent depression. They haven't.[4] Nevertheless, today, the number of these prescriptions has surpassed one million. Psychiatrist Peter Breggin estimates that, each year, 10 percent of the school-age population will take one or more psychiatric drugs.[5] Some children are prescribed several at once. And the phenomenon continues to grow despite disturbing evidence of severe drug-induced personality changes, manic reactions, and psychotic behavior.

Medication advocates would argue that those children who are prescribed psychotropic drugs do in fact need them. Children with affective disturbances or attention deficits can focus better, and thus learn better when medicated, they say. Opponents protest that the efficacy and safety of these drugs have not been proven, and some, further, believe that many psychiatric "conditions" exist only as labels in the minds of psychologists. Whether or not these conditions are real, one must agree that the exceedingly high numbers of prescriptions written for children in recent years are a cause for grave concern. And they're of concern not just to the children and parents directly touched by individual diagnoses, but to society at large. Consider the Columbine massacre and the rash of other school shootings that have rocked this country recently. As the *Washington Times Insight Magazine* reports, "the common link in the high school shootings may be psychotropic drugs like Ritalin and Prozac." For example, in 1998, 14-year-old Kip Kinkle killed his parents and then went on a shooting spree at his Springfield, Oregon, high school, killing two and injuring 22. He was being treated with Ritalin and Prozac. Then there was the15-year-old taking Ritalin who in 1999 wounded six classmates in Heritage High School in Georgia, and the 18-year-old who raped and murdered a 7-year-old girl in 1997, one week after starting to take Dexedrine. One can't help but ask whether psychotropic drugs are dangerous not just to those taking them, but also, in some cases, to "innocent bystanders."

And there are some other basic questions people are beginning to ask as well: Do all these children need to be taking all these drugs? Are they really sick?

By far, the overwhelming majority of psychotropic prescriptions for children are given for attention deficit disorder (ADD) or attention deficit hyperactivity disorder (ADHD). In some instances, taking medicine is a prerequisite for attending school, with refusal to comply considered grounds for dismissal, or worse, removal of the child from the home by the state. This outrages Dr. Fred Baughman, a board-certified child neurologist trained at New York University and Mount Sinai, and a fellow of the American Academy of Neurology. Baughman feels that it's one thing for a court to intervene and take over as legal guardian in a case where a child's life is truly at risk, but quite another thing when psychotropic drugs are forced on children who don't fit into the mold. For instance, Baughman says, for religious reasons parents may refuse a needed blood transfusion for a child, or they may refuse to allow treatment of diabetes—a real disease—with insulin, a real treatment. The courts may have to intervene in such cases. But courts should have no place in mandating that behavioral problems in children be treated with drugs. "There are no physical or chemical abnormalities in these children," Baughman states. "The idea that there is a false belief spouted by psychiatry. . . . For courts to intervene and to mandate such treatment, as though these were legitimate diseases or legitimate medical emergencies, is leading to tyranny over parents of normal children . . . .When we're talking about . . . so-called psychiatric disorders, none of them are actual diseases due to physical abnormalities within the child," states Baughman.[6]

An important argument against the thesis that ADHD and ADD are actual conditions is that the epidemic appears to be confined to North America. The use of Ritalin and similar prescriptions is overwhelmingly concentrated in the United States and Canada. In fact, these two countries account for 96 percent of their use throughout the world, and children in the U.S. have been estimated to be from 10 to 50 times more likely to be labeled as having ADD than their counterparts in Britain or France.[7] In American public schools, about 10 percent of all children in grades K–12 carries an ADHD diagnosis. Europe, by contrast, has a fraction of one percent so labeled. Could the United States and Canada really be so unique in the recent drastic upsurge of this malady?

Many in the health field are calling for more research in this area. For instance, Thomas Moore, senior fellow in health policy at George Washington University Medical Center, who feels that brain damage from Ritalin is more common than has been admitted, often questions the rationale of giving Ritalin to children, stating that the chemical imbalance theory has not been established by any scientific evidence. And while the public is given information by the National Institutes of Mental Health that ADHD is neurobiological in nature, NIMH psychiatrist Peter Jensen stated in 1996, "The National Institutes of Mental Health does not have an official position on whether ADHD is a neurobiological disorder." In other words, this agency is talking out of both sides of its mouth—not that this is an uncommon phenomenon in Washington.

Psychologist Diane McGuiness summed up the situation in 1991 by saying, "We have invented a disease, given it medical sanction, and now must disown it. The major question is, how do we go about destroying the monster we've created? It is not easy to do this and still save face."

Psychologist Daniel Elkind, in his 1981 classic *The Hurried Child,* discussed the increasing "industrialization" of our schools, with their regimented schedules, even at the elementary level, and their focus on turning out quality-controlled products, i.e., students.[8] Today, with administrators under the gun to have their students perform well on standardized tests, and with more troubled children in the schools, the atmosphere has not gotten any more relaxed. The inescapable fact is that schools have an interest in keeping order, in keeping children quiet and calm so they can get on with the business of teaching and learning. And psychiatric medicines do help keep schoolchildren under control. So, in the words of developmental pediatrician Dr. Joseph Keeley, "We sometimes use medications to make kids fit into schools rather than schools to fit the kids."[9]

Of course there are better ways to make schools work, such as appropriate therapy for troubled youngsters, custom-tailored education plans, and small classes. But these approaches are more difficult—and more expensive. Thus, the school district may have a vested interest in medication as a quick, less costly, fix, although this may not be what's best for a particular child. Says Dr. David Stein, "The drugs blunt their behavior. They don't act out in class, and they sit there quietly . . . .The difficulty is that children learn nothing from a drug."[10]

Schools justify the need for medications by saying that children on Ritalin learn better because the drug allows them to focus, but that claim has never been proven. According to Stein, so-called ADD children can learn when they want to; it's just that schools expect too much of students and do not engage them. "This country has started teaching second- and third-grade material in kindergarten, and children begin to get burnt out by the time they're in the second grade. They wind up hating schoolwork. And that's the key. These children can play very complex video games, and they can read the instructions, because they enjoy doing it."[11]

The situation in American schools today was chillingly illustrated for me by a teacher I talked with recently. She works for a state-funded organization that sends teachers, social workers, psychologists, and speech therapists to disadvantaged schools for support. Once a week, she explained, there are meetings with the principal, other staff, and sometimes parents to discuss specific problem children. "Although we are given no specific training in how to advise or function as a team," she said, "we are looked at as experts, and our advice is highly regarded. In my experience, the meetings are merely attempts to find quick-fix solutions, and since the psychologist dominates, the answer to a great many childhood problems is an ADHD or ADD diagnosis for which medication is considered the logical solution."

This teacher told me she will never forget an experience she had when she was fairly new to team meetings. "After another teacher had expressed concern about an active second grader, the psychologist and psychology intern reported their findings to the parents at a team meeting. They said that the boy fit the ADHD profile because he had gotten out of his seat so many times in class and couldn't sit still without fidgeting. They suggested that he should be taken to a doctor for follow-up.

"The mother initially asked an intelligent question: 'Will the doctor perform a special kind of test to determine that my son has a medical disorder?' The team could not answer that question in the affirmative since no such test is performed. The doctor merely observes the child's behavior, looks at the behavior checklist filled out by the parent and teacher, and then fills out a prescription.

"While the mother appeared immediately receptive to persuasion, the quiet father wore an expression of concern in his eyes. The principal asked what was wrong, and the father responded in one word: 'Ritalin.' The team then turned their attention to soothing the father, saying that medication would be in the boy's best interest because once he was calm he would be able to pay attention to his schoolwork and succeed in his studies."

When the meeting ended, the teacher said, she pulled the father aside and told him that she understood his concerns. "I told him that many parents were opposed to medicating their children and that alternative approaches did exist. Then I handed him a brochure on alternative approaches." She felt she had to take a discreet approach because she'd learned, from past meetings, that it was useless to speak up. The psychologists are so married to their ideology that they're quick to shoot down the opposition. "Even though I attempted to be confidential," she reported, "the room was small, and I could feel the psychologist's eyes glaring at me, as if she was going to use the information to report me to the thought-control police."

Once the parent's left, the teacher went on to relate, the red-faced principal exclaimed, "That burns me up! Here we are trying so hard to help their son, and the father gives us a hard time." Obviously, the principal did not understand why the idea of medicating a young child, possibly every single day for the rest of his life, should concern parents.

Soon after that, the parents complied. The next time this teacher saw the second-grader in her math group, he was already on Ritalin, so she was able to see a before-and-after contrast in personality. The child had been a bit antsy before, calling out or even getting out of his seat from time to time, but his behavior seemed normal. Now the child seemed severely depressed. He would cry for the smallest slight, losing a turn in a board game, for example, and even crawl under the table to cry. He had never acted that way before. On one occasion he told the teacher that he wanted to kill himself. She reported that to the psychologist, who seemed annoyed at the trouble. Soon the psychologist reported back to the teacher that the parents didn't notice any difference in behavior. He would continue as before.

This teacher went on to make the point that biological "treatments" for childhood social disorders are not discriminatory; i.e., she has seen the same arrogance and insensitivity in an affluent school district on the other side of town. In the high school where she worked as a reading specialist, teachers confronted with children they deem problematic routinely say to peers and parents, "He [or she] should be on meds." The students' perceived problems can range from inability to focus to acting out to just not being able to read. At one meeting, highly educated parents of a very bright young lady with reading difficulties were looking for a specific diagnosis to work with and were told by the psychologist to consider seeing a doctor about her daughter's possible ADD— attention deficit disorder without the hyperactivity component. To the teacher's relief, the parents glanced at each other, snickering to themselves, as if to say, "I can't believe you would say such a thing."

If only more parents would laugh in the face of this absurdity. Some parents do seem aware of the ADD controversy, but overall there is blind acceptance of ADD as a true medical condition and of medication as a requirement.

It should be noted that it's not just elementary and high schools that seem to need a drug to help them run smoothly, but preschools and day care centers also. As writer Robyn Suriano recently pointed out in the *Orlando Sentinel*,[12] "The drug [Ritalin] reached its heyday in the 1990s, after more children started attending day care. In a preschool, kids must follow instructions and behave just like older children in classrooms. Rambunctious ones are not easily tolerated in these surroundings, where workers must watch many children." This is not to say that day care centers are necessarily bad, but there are a lot of inadequately staffed and equipped ones. These trap preschoolers in confining, boring situations for 10 hours a day and then complain when they act like the active, inquisitive, and needy young creatures that children just barely out of babyhood normally are. That drugs are used to remedy this situation is unconscionable, especially considering that Ritalin's label warns that the drug is only for those aged 6 and over. But "off-label" prescription is legal, and it's happening. As a *Wall Street Journal* article reported,[13] the use of prescription drugs to control toddlers' behavior has increased dramatically in the past decade.

The *Journal* article did give voice to a couple of dissenting professionals concerning this trend. Psychiatrist Joseph Coyle, chairman of the Department of Psychiatry at Harvard Medical School, was one. The brains of young children are developing rapidly, he pointed out, and drugs can alter the process. Coyle also cited the financial interests of managed care in creating a system in which doctors are too busy to do much more than prescribe. And Dr. Julie Zito, an associate professor at the University of Maryland's School of Pharmacy, was especially skeptical of the use of Ritalin to combat attention-deficit disorder in two-year-olds. "What is abnormally inattentive in a two-year-old?" she asked.

It was Dr. Zito who, along with colleagues from the University of Maryland, Johns Hopkins, and Kaiser Permanente's Center for Health Research, authored a study on "Trends in the Prescribing of Psychotropic Medications to Preschoolers."[14] Published in the *Journal of the American Medical Association*, the study contained some unsettling findings concerning very young children and psychotropic drugs. The researchers found that poor—and particularly black—children are being prescribed Ritalin at younger and younger ages. A 300-percent increase in prescriptions to the very young between 1991 and 1995 was cited. The study also mentioned Prozac being given to children younger than one year of age, to the tune of some 3000 prescriptions in 1994.

Before ADD and ADHD came into vogue, amphetamines were seldom prescribed. Ritalin was given for narcolepsy, a rare neurological disorder that causes people to fall asleep unexpectedly despite adequate sleep, but sales were minuscule. Now, thanks to the popularity of ADD and ADHD, Ritalin sales are significantly healthier. Moreover, the psychiatric establishment has seemingly discovered several other childhood disorders, including pediatric depression, for which medications are routinely prescribed. By the way, most of the people prescribing psychiatric drugs are not psychiatrists, but primary-care physicians, who have not received the kind of sophisticated mental-health training needed to understand what's involved in prescribing these life-altering substances. Our managed-care system of health care bears at least some of the blame for this trend. As a recent article in *Parents* magazine point out, "Here, as with almost everything else in the tangled world of health care, economics plays a decisive role. Drugs have become the treatment of first resort when kids exhibit behavioral problems, partly because most managed-care plans readily cover the cost of medication but often won't pay for long-term alternative treatments, such as talk or behavioral therapy."[15]

The people who manage managed care are not particularly interested in getting to the source of patients' problems, focused as they are on the bottom line and the quick fix. Psychiatrist Dr. David Kaiser elaborates: "When I talk to a managed care representative about the care of one of my patients, they invariably want to know about medications I am using and little else, and there is often an implication that I am not medicating aggressively enough. There is now a growing cottage industry within psychiatry in advocating ways to work with managed care, despite the obvious fact that managed care has little interest in quality care and realistic approaches to real patients. This financial pressure by managed care contributes added pressure for psychiatry to go down a biological road and to avoid more realistic treatment approaches."[16]

The boom in psychiatric drug sales has been helped along by a vigorous marketing campaign. Psychiatrist Loren Mosher reports that at meetings of the American Psychiatric Association, drug companies "basically lease 90 percent of the exhibition space and spend huge sums in giveaway items. They have nearly completely squeezed out the little guys, and the symposiums that once were dedicated to scientific reports now have been replaced by the pharmaceutical-industry-sponsored speakers."[17] And pitches for drugs are made not just to medical practitioners, but also to teachers and parents. In the early 1990s, pharmaceutical companies distributed pamphlets to schools nationwide on how to diagnose ADHD and ADD, conditions for which medication was presented as the solution. During this time America saw a dramatic rise in Ritalin consumption, close to a 700-percent increase. Ritalin's manufacturer also funded CHADD to encourage parents to support the drug solution and to keep public confidence levels high. Today, drug companies continue to spend hundreds of thousands of advertising dollars in psychiatric journals.

They've also started advertising in popular magazines. Recently, some stimulant manufacturers have gone against standard international practice and begun marketing directly to parents. Here's how *The New York Times* describes this appalling trend:[18]

* * *

"In the back-to-school section of this month's [Aug. 2001] *Ladies' Home Journal*, tucked among the ads for Life cereal, bologna and Jell-O pudding, are three full-page advertisements for the A.D.H.D. treatments.

"The ads evoke a sense of Rockwellian calm. Children chat happily next to a school bus. A child's hand gently touches the hand of an adult. In one, for the new drug Metadate CD, an approving mother embraces her beaming son as the drug itself is named and promoted.

"This is a first. Metadate CD, like Ritalin, Adderall and similar drugs, are what are known as Schedule II controlled substances, the most addictive substances that are still legal. (Schedule I drugs like heroin and LSD are illegal.)

"In keeping with a 1971 international treaty, such controlled substances have never been marketed directly to consumers, only to doctors. There is, however, no federal law to prevent drug companies from doing it . . . .The new magazine advertisement by Celltech Pharmaceuticals, the British maker of Metadate CD, states, 'Introducing Metadate capsules. One dose covers his A.D.H.D. for the whole school day.' "

According to *The Times*, in the year 2000 close to 20 million prescriptions were written for ADD medicines, with sales bringing in about $758 million. It is true that a lot of this profit goes into research that tests drugs' safety and efficacy. The obvious down side to this, though, is that with companies funding their own testing, results can be biased, as it is not in a company's best interest to get negative results that discourage business.

This conflict-of-interest situation raises ethical issues that are especially troublesome when you consider that it is children who are being targeted by these drug companies. Furthermore, today it's not just the classic "problem child" who is being targeted for stimulant consumption. As Peter Breggin points out in *Talking Back to Ritalin,*[19] there is a wide range of children being given stimulants, from the truly hyperactive child who can't sit still for a second to the child without severe behavior problems who is simply dreamy or inattentive. As is the case with other psychotropics, the net of this drug's reach seems to have widened.

Many children taking Ritalin will develop involuntary muscle contractions and limb movements known as tics, or dyskinesia. A study published in the *Archives of Pediatric and Adolescent Medicine*[20] showed that this can happen to up to 9 percent of children taking stimulants. Other studies in the peer-reviewed medical literature bear out this association,[21,22,23] as well as the Ritalin-psychosis connection. Also, Ritalin has also been shown to have an adverse effect on heart tissue and has been linked to cancer. In the mid-90s, the FDA forced Ritalin's maker to send letters to 100,000 doctors, warning them of a possible link between the drug and liver cancer. Researchers reported to the FDA that their studies show "clear evidence" that link the drug to cancer. The FDA changed the warning to "some evidence," a change that was protested by one of the main researchers. A formal proposal to keep the wording "clear evidence" was presented to an FDA panel, but this was defeated by a vote of 4 to 3. "Clear evidence" became "some evidence," and ultimately the FDA publicly announced that there was "a weak link" between Ritalin and cancer and that doctors should not be concerned about continuing to prescribe the drug.

A problem that some children and teenagers experience with Ritalin is called rebound. When the drug is metabolized and the level in the bloodstream goes down, these children seem to go back to a hyperactive state "and then some." They may get excitable or impulsive, or develop insomnia.[24] In fact, as many as half the so-called ADHD children on medications report some presleep agitation, called P-A.[25] Physicians try to handle this problem by decreasing the last dose of the day, or, alternatively, adding another dose, so that the child sleeps with a new supply of Ritalin in his blood. Sometimes this works, but one has to wonder about the advisability of children taking a sleep-pattern-altering drug over the long term.

Yet another Ritalin side effect is the stunting of growth that occurs in some children taking moderate to high stimulant dosages over a period of years. This happens not just because stimulants can diminish appetite, but also because they may alter the body's natural balance of growth hormones.[26]The growth-stunting phenomenon doesn't seem to have alarmed the medical establishment as much as it should. Consider the advice given by clinical psychologist Dr. John Taylor in his book *Helping Your Hyperactive/Attention Deficit Child*.[27] The author notes, first, that some physicians recommend taking the child off medication during vacation periods, so that he can catch up in height and weight. Then Taylor counsels: "The crucial question is whether your child's behavior can be tolerated if he or she is unmedicated (or undermedicated) during the summer months. Several adjustments are available. Your child can play outdoors more, attend camps, participate in athletic programs or other vigorous play activities, or even be sent to live with a relative. There is little or no requirement for intense academic pursuits, there is no need to sit still for hours as is required in school, and summer entertainments can take advantage of your child's interests to prevent boredom . . . .Among those who are not given any medication-free periods and who experience the stunting effect, the average amount is less than two inches. If stunting occurs and becomes an important psychological issue, choice of hair style and footwear can compensate."

At least three questions arise. First, if it's possible to give a child a stimulating and active life in the summer, at camp or with relatives, why can't this be done in the winter, in school and with the nuclear family? Surely arranging for more outdoor playtime, and more interesting activities, is preferable to putting a child on drugs. Second, do parents and doctors have the right to stunt a child's growth for any reason other than, perhaps, to save his life? And third, even if "choice of hair style and footwear can compensate," for decreased height, how is the child going to feel about this later, when he understands what's been done to him?

In addition to all the potentially damaging effects of Ritalin one has to factor in the reality that it doesn't work. Yes, it does make some children better behaved at certain times. But there are no studies showing improved academic performance or social behavior over the long term.[28] What *has* been shown over the long term is that the side effects can become quite serious.

Most people assume that drugs are proven safe before they are marketed. But this is not always the case, especially when you consider the long-term picture. Science knows very little about the long-term effects of medicating children. In effect, children have been guinea pigs. The results of this grand experiment are only now becoming evident, and sometimes the consequences are deadly.

Consider the case of Stephanie Hall, a first grader placed on Ritalin because her teacher felt she was "just a little bit too antsy," according to her mother. "[The teacher] suggested that Stephanie go for testing, so we went the route of a neurologist who said she could throw a ball and read a book and a psychologist who said she had average intelligence but, yes, she was a little easily distracted. So now she qualifies to be medicated." When she turned 12, the prescription was increased; that very day, Stephanie died from cardiac arrest in her sleep. Says her mom, "Her death was caused by cardiac arrhythmia with no family history of any type of heart problem whatsoever, and she died a day after her medicine had been increased. It kind of adds up."[29]

A double tragedy struck the Hall family when Stephanie's sister Jenny, also a long-term Ritalin user, started to have seizures. Subsequent medical tests revealed a brain tumor. Mrs. Hall believes that Jenny was misdiagnosed; as a result proper medical attention was delayed. She states, "There's Jenny's ADHD, it's a brain tumor. I'm not saying everyone that is labeled ADHD has a brain tumor. . . . But there's the possibility that a child could have an underlying neurological disease that really needs treatment." Mrs. Hall also wonders whether the medication could have precipitated or exacerbated Jenny's condition: "It probably made her condition worse because prior to being on medication she never had seizures. I later read that if you have a low threshold to seizures you should never take Ritalin to begin with."[30] She and her husband are suing Novartis, the maker of Ritalin, for producing a defective product and concealing adverse reactions and deaths related to its use.[31]

The once trusting mother advises parents to learn from her mistakes: "Don't trust your doctor. Question him over and over. If you are not happy with what he says, if you have an intuitive feeling that something doesn't seem right, it's not. Get second and third opinions. It may not seem reasonable to have to go to that extent, but if it's at the price of your child, it is. I hope others can learn from my tragedy and realize that a doctor's word is not God's law."[32]

In a more publicized story, Matthew Smith, a 14-year-old from

Michigan, had also, like Stephanie Hall, been taking Ritalin from the time he was in first grade. After eight years of ingesting the drug daily, Matthew suddenly became pulseless and died while riding his scooter. An autopsy performed by the county medical examiner, a Dr. Dragovic, found that Matthew's heart muscle was diffusely replaced with scar tissue, as were the muscular walls of the coronary vessels. Much to the displeasure of the psychiatric and pharmaceutical industry, the doctor publicly stated that Matthew's death was undoubtedly due to heart damage akin to that regularly seen in deaths among amphetamine addicts, and that his death was clearly due to the Ritalin.

Yet another incident occurred in a psychiatric facility near San Antonio, Texas, where young Randy Steele was being restrained when he suddenly died. Randy was on several psychiatric drugs at the time. But his first psychiatric diagnosis, his entry into a life of psychiatry, had been ADHD, and his first drug was Dexedrine or dextroamphetamine. At death he had an enlarged heart.

It should surprise no one to learn that Ritalin and other amphetamines can lead to death. The dangers are well known to doctors who study the adverse effects of these substances as medical students. Dr. Dragovic explains: "Methylphenidate— that's [Ritalin's] chemical name—is classified as an adrenergic agonist. This is a type of drug that boosts the adrenergic system. It affects everything that has as its chemical pathway adrenalin, noradrenaline, dopamine, those types of mediators and transmitters. Drugs in the category of stimulants also include Ritalin's cousins—amphetamines, methamphetamines, and even cocaine. If they are repetitively used, these drugs stimulate the adrenergic system in the human body. Over a period of time . . . many months to many years—the enhancement of the adrenergic system will produce changes in small blood vessels. Some cells will be lost, and in an attempt to repair the area there will be scarring . . . .The blood vessels will narrow. The changes that we're seeing in kids who have been on Ritalin for about eight years are basically the same as the changes in someone that has been abusing cocaine regularly over a period of years."[33]

Dragovic adds that irreversible damage to the vascular system could also result in cardiovascular problems down the road, including high blood pressure. By medicating vast numbers of children today, we could be creating an army of future patients with other conditions that need to be treated. "Do we need that?" asks Dr. Dragovic. His answer is certainly no, but as he explains, "That's the peril of chronic Ritalin use, or of any stimulant for that matter. It's paying the due to long-term use."[34]

There are few if any statistics on how many people experience adverse effects. What we do know is that, according to FDA adverse reaction reports—which are notoriously incomplete— there were 160 Ritalin-related deaths between 1990 and 1997, most of them cardiovascular-related. We know that Ritalin is a vasoactive (blood-vessel-altering) substance that decreases cerebral blood flow.[35] And we know that children's brains are undergoing dramatic development through the teen years, not just in early childhood, as had been previously thought.[36] We also know that Ritalin can have persistent, cumulative effects on the myocardium, the muscle cells that form most of the heart wall.[37] With all these facts in mind, one has to wonder about the implications for the millions of American children being dosed over the long term with stimulants. As Dr. Fred Baughman points out, "There is no way of knowing the actual frequency of . . . any medical side effects of these drugs, because there is no required reporting system. There is only a voluntary system whereby physicians would call the FDA, and, needless to say, they don't often report their own complications."[38] Ritalin's vast growth—its legal and illegal use—could mean that a multitude of tragedies are on the horizon.

There are those who believe that what we perceive as ADHD is simply children's natural reaction to the sped-up quality of much of American life today. One of these people is psychologist Dr. Richard DeGrandpre, fellow of the National Institute on Drug Abuse and author of *Ritalin Nation*.[39] "As society goes faster, so do the rhythms of our own consciousness," DeGrandpre writes in this insightful book.[40] "This is especially true for children, who grow up in concert with the latest speed." DeGrandpre points out that young people who have known nothing but a hurried, perpetually wired environment, will tend to get restless when the stimulation level lags—in a classroom, for instance. And he says that Ritalin, being itself a stimulant, does not so much erase the need for excitement but rather fulfill it, in a prosthetic way. Indeed, he coins the phrase "prosthetic pharmacology" to refer to the way modern psychiatry uses drugs as crutches, rather than cures. And while a real crutch may help a person's injured leg heal, psychiatric crutches often mask underlying problems, resulting in no effort being made to deal with them.

A noteworthy point made by DeGrandpre is that, while years ago, the condition then known as hyperactivity tended to disappear when childhood ended, today's ADHD seems to linger into adolescence and adulthood for a lot of its "victims." But why would a bona fide disorder suddenly afflict a whole new age group? There has to be a cultural component at play.

We don't seem to want to face any cultural concerns, though. We'd rather diagnose a large segment of the population as mentally impaired, thereby shifting responsibility for our mental well-being away from society and toward the medical profession. When people are identified as "sick," their issues are seen as the result of a diseased mind, rather than as a reaction to an unhealthy family dynamic or social environment. But one need only compare the world of today to that of 50 years ago to appreciate the magnitude of the additional stresses in contemporary times that could result in maladaptive behavior. Many children practically grow up in day care centers, for example, their parents being too busy and hassled to raise them, and dinner is usually eaten in front of the TV. Family members don't interact with each other. School demands more academic work from children at an earlier age. The extended family is practically nonexistent, with grandparents, aunts, and uncles living many states away. As a result, values are not taught to children. The divorce rate is approaching 67 percent, and 50 percent of children are being raised by single parents. These statements about modern life are almost cliché, but the fact remains that the environment they describe does have an impact on children.

I believe you have to look deeply at the values of a society to really understand what ails its people. In today's America, it never occurs to anyone that it's okay to just be by being. In our society we hate the idea of being without purpose. Baby boomers, in particular, feel that we're always supposed to have a purpose, a goal, a motivation to get there, discipline to keep the motivation going, and passion to fuel it all. We're supposed to have a higher ideal, and to value success and competition. But in the process of doing all that we frequently lose our sense of identity. We have to consider that when today's kids take a careful look at their parents, they may not want to duplicate what they see. They—or at least some of them—may be turned off by the high stress levels, the judgmental attitudes, the lack of quality of life, the lack of unconditional love, the absence of peace of mind, and the inability to feel comfortable with what is. So kids may say, "I'm just going to kind of hang out in the moment." And we think, "No, you can't. You've got to get in there. You've got to achieve. You've got to prove yourself. You're up against competition. There's a shortage of everything." And then we put them in a situation where they can't win and can only be labeled as having some kind of deficit.

An alien observer looking at the current drug situation in the United States would certainly be confused. On the one hand we're preaching drug avoidance to our youth. On the other, we're dosing a lot of them with mind-altering drugs, which, as we've just seen, can sometimes be tragically behavior altering as well.

One of the results of our eagerness to fix problems with drugs is the widespread abuse of drugs that have been legally prescribed to children. According to the DEA, Ritalin and other stimulants are among the most frequently stolen prescription medicines,[41] with the pills often crushed and snorted for an immediate high. Ritalin is now a prime choice among the drugs abused on college campuses across the country. High school students use it recreationally as well. A 1997 Indiana University survey reported that nearly 7 percent of high school students had engaged in this practice.[42]

It's time to reassess what we want for our children. Do we want to bring them up in a drug culture or not? Do we want to mold them into the confines of our educational system, or do we want to fashion an education that will respond to *their* needs? What are our criteria for a successful child? And will we continue to label those who don't meet these criteria as psychologically abnormal? We're sticking this label onto an awful lot of kids lately.

An important point was made in *Contemporary Directions in Psychopathology*, a textbook used to train psychiatrists.[43] It was stated that there was "evidence that the current psychiatric diagnosis system is a reflection of social, cultural developments rather than scientific data." The editor of this book, Gerald Clerman, also edited *The Archives of General Psychiatry*, and sat on the American Psychiatric Association's task force for its diagnostic and statistical manual of mental disorders, the "psychiatrist's bible" of diagnostic labels. So basically, in a totally "establishment" textbook, we have an admission that social and cultural expectations, rather than objective science, form the basis for the way we evaluate who is mentally abnormal.

We would do well to remember this—and then to rethink our penchant for labeling—before we prescribe any more brain-altering drugs to children.

In light of our theme that the mental-health industry is pathologizing life–a very broad category, then we would have to look at the other end of its spectrum, the elderly, to see if our argument applies.

A woman in her 70 copes with recurring bouts of depression after the death of her beloved husband. She consults a psychiatrist who tells her all she needs to bring her out of the dark is ECT, electroconvulsive therapy. What he fails to consider is that his patient has a weak heart, and the consent form she signs mentions nothing of this risk. The woman allows herself to undergo treatment and, days later, dies.

This particular scenario is made up, but variations on it happen all too frequently. Consider that half the 100,000 Americans being shocked each year are senior citizens. Now consider records from Texas, the only state required to track complications within two weeks of ECT administration. These records document a death rate from ECT of 1 in 200 recipients of the treatment. Statistics also reveal that the typical candidate for ECT is a depressed middle- or upper-middle-class woman in her 70s who checks herself into a private hospital. The targeted population has shifted since the 1950s and '60s, when schizophrenic men in their 40s were the primary group subjected to ECT, and the reason is economics. Insurance no longer supports long hospital stays, but Medicare, the government's medical insurance program for people 65 and older, will generously reimburse psychiatrists who administer ECT. This incentive is apparent once again in Texas records, which show 65-year-olds receiving 360 percent more shock therapy than 64-year-olds.[44]

But paralleling the growth of ECT is the growing number of critics of the treatment, both within and outside of the psychiatric establishment. Shock is not just ineffective, the opposition claims, it often leaves recipients in a worsened condition than before treatment. Depression and suicidal ideation soon return, complicated by ECT-induced brain damage and memory loss. Plus new conditions, such as epilepsy and heart arrhythmias, can develop. Moreover, signing the permission form for this treatment may be signing your life away, as the risk of death during or soon after the procedure is great, far higher than ECT proponents admit, in part due to the targeting of fragile elderly populations. ECT's most ardent challengers, often former patients themselves, wonder how healing professionals could have forgotten their Hippocratic oath to do no harm. They assert that ECT is a barbaric procedure that must be banned.

But why has ECT had a revival? Consider that sixty years ago, once ECT was adopted in the U.S., abuse of this modality became common. This is not to say that the treatment is not in and of itself an abuse, but from the 1940s to the '70s, shock treatments were often given in psychiatric hospitals not just as treatment, but to quiet or punish patients. Notes one woman I interviewed, of her experience in the early '70s: "I wasn't depressed; I wasn't suicidal . . . . They were shocking everyone on the ward—the young, the really old, everyone. . . . What were they shocking us for? . . . Ward control?" Medical historian David J. Rothman of Columbia University points out that ECT stands practically alone among medical/surgical interventions in its role as a patient control mechanism used for the benefit of the hospital staff."[45]

Economic factors of the 1980s brought ECT into the limelight once again, particularly insurance policies that refused to pay for lengthy therapies but readily reimbursed short-term hospital procedures like ECT. Since then, electroshock has received glowing endorsements from numerous organizations, including the National Institutes of Health, the National Alliance for the Mentally Ill, the National Depressive and Manic Depressive Association, and the American Psychological Association. This last organization takes an active role in ECT advocacy. This includes fighting attempts to restrict the procedure, and working to relax current standards so that shock therapy will become an initial, rather than last-resort, treatment for the depressed.[46]

Although present-day modifications can help in certain ways by reducing a patient's fear and stopping flailing movements that can cause bone fractures, the treatment itself—the zapping of the brain with an electrical current—is the same as it has been, and inevitably results in brain damage. According to the National Head Injury Foundation, each treatment equals one moderate-to-severe head injury.[47] And as a series of shocks are prescribed—eight to fifteen on average and as many as one per month on an indefinite basis—the wounding intensifies. In 1983, Dr. Sydney Samant described what happens in the following way: "As a neurologist and electroencephalographer, I have seen many patients after ECT, and I have no doubt that ECT produces effects identical to those of a head injury. After multiple sessions of ECT, a patient has symptoms identical to those of a retired, punch-drunk boxer. . . . After a few sessions of ECT the symptoms are those of moderate cerebral contusion, and further enthusiastic use of ECT may result in the patient functioning at a subhuman level. Electroconvulsive therapy, in effect, may be defined as a controlled type of brain damage produced by electrical means."[48]

The scientific literature is replete with research confirming memory damage from ECT as the rule rather than the exception. For example, in Freeman and Kendell's 1986 study, 74 percent of patients mentioned "memory impairment" as a continuing problem, and "a striking 30 percent felt that their memory had been permanently affected." The authors mentioned that these symptoms were probably under-reported because the patients were interviewed by the same doctors who treated them.[49] An interesting note: The 1990 APA task force cites Freeman and Kendell— these same authors—as indicating, "a small minority of patients, however, report persistent deficits."

Cardiovascular complications arising out of ECT are commonly seen in the scientific literature. For instance, the *Journal of Clinical Psychiatry* reported that 28 percent of a group of 42 patients undergoing ECT suffered cardiovascular problems following treatment. Of the patients who already had a history or indication of cardiac disease, 70 percent developed cardiac complications."[50] The *Journal of Humanistic Psychology* reported on a 57-year-old man who died of heart rupture after receiving several shock treatments."[51] From that same article: "Physicians from Tulane University Medical School reported on a 69-year-old woman who developed brain hemorrhage during ECT. She was also left with epilepsy afterward. This was, as expected, associated with further deterioration in her mental status from her baseline depression. They conclude that the fragile vessels of the elderly may make some patients a particularly high risk for ECT."

Psychiatrists hail electroshock as the best method for curing affective disorders and stopping suicides. One of its most zealous proponents, Dr. Max Fink, a professor of psychiatry at the State University of New York at Stony Brook and the editor-in-chief of *Convulsive Therapy,* goes so far as to proclaim ECT "God's gift to man" and has stated that "[it should be given to] all patients whose condition is severe enough to require hospitalization."[52, 53] A closer look, however, casts doubt on psychiatry's enthusiasm. To begin, one needs to ask what psychiatrists actually mean when they call electroshock effective. For how long do patients show improvement from depression? What do studies conclude about ECT and suicide prevention? And what do psychiatrists actually consider patient improvement?

What an ECT fact sheet fails to tell patients is that improvements are temporary. Studies have never concluded that patients remain depression-free for longer than a month.[54] Initially, ECT recipients score higher on the Hamilton depression scale, a test used to measure depression, but weeks later their scores drop again. This is why psychiatrists recommend follow-up treatments with antidepressants or more electroshock every few weeks. Maintenance with antidepressants, however, does not guarantee success, according to one study published in the *New England Journal of Medicine.* The study reported a 59–percent return to depression two months following ECT.[55]

Electroconvulsive therapy is to psychiatry what open-heart surgery and hysterectomy are to other branches of medicine—a lucrative income booster. Charges of several hundreds of dollars per treatment add up quickly, so that physicians shocking patients three times a week, for instance, can increase their salary by over $27,000 a year,[56] and more ambitious doctors may receive a $200,000 bonus.[57] With the electroshock industry grossing two to three billion dollars a year, and psychiatric groups lobbying for relaxed restrictions, doctors have ample opportunity for financial gain.[58]

Since most insurance policies permit month-long hospital stays, a course of ECT may be begun right away. Or it may start a month later when Major Medical insurance kicks in for "major" treatment protocols, of which ECT is one. This second option is the best deal for private psychiatric facilities (where the bulk of ECT takes place), as beds remain filled longer for a charge of several thousand dollars per patient. Afterwards, insurance will reimburse patients for outpatient follow-up procedures, in which people are drugged, shocked, wheeled into the recovery room while in a coma, and sent home in a stupor the very same day. The importance of insurance in influencing who gets treatment was noted by one psychiatrist, who stated, "Finding that the patient has insurance seemed like the most common indication for giving electroshock."[59]

The fact is that anyone speaking to a psychiatrist is at risk of being perceived as psychopathological. All a psychiatrist need do is pick one or more conditions that seem to fit from the psychiatric "bible," the DSM manual, where hundreds of so-called "diagnosable conditions" are listed—everything from insomnia, worry, and caffeinism, to being shy. Very few of the "disorders" are organic; the majority are socially based.

In its rush to diagnose and treat, what psychiatry forgets is that mental symptoms can be caused by poor physical health. An example of misdiagnosis is the case of Ruth Reed Price, whose nervous breakdown resulted in a diagnosis of schizophrenia when the real problem, discovered later, was a thyroid imbalance. In her 1995 testimony on banning electric shock in Austin, Texas, Price talked of the damage to her memory and nervous system that made returning to work a nightmare. "Instead of trying to really discover what was wrong," she says, "the Austin State Hospital staff made a wrong assumption and preceded to damage my brain and impair my memory with their violent electric shock therapy."

So, one of the effects of the new pathologizing of life itself today is that older technologies, even disgraced ones like ECT, are retrieved as the arsenal for this panicked invasion of our bodies must be expanded since newer alternative modalities that do not stigmatize normal life experiences must be avoided.

The present misguided and exploitative policies in health care regarding depression and schizophrenia also have the dispiriting effect of continuing anti-social traditions like racism. The irony is that long-standing social pathologies of past cultures and social groupings have a renewed "life" because they become ad hoc justifications within the larger agenda of pathologizing life. For example, what we see happening in the African American community today has, in the minds of many, been created: blacks-against-blacks violence, suicide and drug abuse at an all time high, children who cannot read or write and a very high level of unemployment. Psychiatrists involuntarily commit African Americans three to five times as often as they do whites. Psychiatrists diagnose African American men in public and private mental hospitals as having schizophrenia at a rate of up to 1,500 percent higher than white men. African Americans are given significantly higher doses of psychiatric drugs, major tranquilizers, and neuroleptics than are whites. More than twice as many African Americans as whites are classified as mentally retarded. Psychiatry—heavily financed by the National Institutes of Mental Health along with this Community Mental Health Centers Program, which began in 1963—has been, in the minds of many, destructive in the oppression of the African Americans. Community health centers have provided numerous frontline sales outlets operating within the fabric of society, entrapping greater numbers of unwitting victims. The growth of this network parallels the declining statistics among African Americans.

William, a young African American, provokes a stark example of the psychiatric approach to mental health. William lost his job and was worried about how he was going to support himself. He could not write. He could not read. He visited a local community mental health center to talk to someone about it. Instead of listening to him, the psychiatrist asked stereotypical questions about whether he abused his girlfriend and if he felt angry. Well this frustrated him. He raised his voice. Within minutes, the psychiatrist had called in two men to involuntarily admit William to a psychiatric institution. He was held for three days against his will, and was forcibly injected with major tranquilizers. For the first two days the main question asked of William was do you have any insurance. He was told that if he wanted help he would need to pay for it. William had no money. Two hours later psychiatrists interviewed him and suddenly found he was fit to be released. Before being discharged, William was told to sign a paper that he could not read. He was later told that this form indemnified the hospital. It said that he had been fully informed about the drugs prescribed to him and he had been willingly able to take them. This is not an isolated case. It is typical of how easy it has been for psychiatrists using diagnostic procedures and repressive mental health laws to incarcerate African Americans.

After World War II, the National Institutes of Mental Health was formed and most of the US psychiatric research had been carried out since 1948 has been funded by The National Institutes of Mental Health. This has included LSD studies being carried out on African American inmates. The 1970's Violence Initiative was planned to isolate African American leaders among inner city youth, and give them psychosurgery or lobotomies to curb "violent behavior." In the 1992, "Violence Initiative" was planned to find "violence causing genes in African American children which can be controlled by powerful psychotropic mind-altering drugs."

In 1992 The National Institutes of Mental Health launched a lucrative plan under the bogus title of Violence Initiative to identify "problem black children." In reality it was to be an experiment on minority races using psychiatric drugs. It was to cost $50 million of taxpayers' money until stopped by groups such as The National Committee Against Federal Violence Initiative. At the time the director of the agency over The National Institutes of Mental Health, psychiatrist Frederick Goodwin, became infamous because of his racist reasoning behind the proposed research that inner city youth are like violent "oversexed Rhesus monkeys in the jungle." When I was researching this I wanted to see surely the Black Caucus and surely some of the black legislator and surely some of the liberal involvement in 1992 would have stopped this. No. To the contrary. The White House fully supported it. The president supported it. The president's wife supported it. I always find it of interest when people go saying they care about you. They suffer for you. They feel for you. You trust that. Then they are part of the group that are behind the idea that you are like a bunch of oversexed Rhesus monkeys that need psychiatric drugs to keep in line. Connect the dots and see if it changes perspective.

What we have is Big Brother as a biological psychiatrist. Even more outlandish possibilities for social and political applications are raised in The Tribune series. For example, monkey research allegedly demonstrated that the more dictatorial leaders have low serotonin while more democratic monkeys had high normal serotonin. Subordinate monkeys supposedly become friendly democratic leaders after being given Prozac. The leap to drugs as a solution for widespread social problems raised the specter of Big Brother as a biological psychiatrist.

African American adolescents between the ages of 13 and 17 are far more likely to be coerced through a mental health center than whites. Forty-six percent of African American adolescents referred to these centers are between 16 and 17. African Americans are twice as likely as whites to enter community mental health centers through a referral agency. From a social agency, 90 percent of the adolescents entering the community mental health system are poor. An August 1998 study on arrest rates of patients at a community mental health center indicates that people attending these centers are nearly two times more likely to be arrested than the general population. Studies show that 55 percent of outpatients visiting a community mental health center receive a psychiatric drug. Summary: As Dr. Thomas Oz says, "The engine that drives the psychiatric industry today is a combination of federal and state funds, government mandated insurance coverage, commitment laws, and the threat of involuntary mental hospitalization together with false claims about effectiveness of neuroleptic drugs."

The forces that actually propelled the change were economic and legal. It was specifically the transfer of funding from psychiatric services from the states to the federal government, and the shift in legal psychiatric fashions from long term drugging. No one in authority challenged the assumptions on which this alleged reform rested. No one asked if it was true that mental illness is like any other illness or if psychiatric drugs made the patient mentally healthier and economically more self-sufficient. On the contrary, careers in politics, psychiatric academia, and the media are made by not asking such questions. Pretending instead that we knew the answers and were there with a resounding yes. The familiar psychiatric code words—such as mental illness, hospital treatment, and schizophrenia—thus remained intact and were fortified with a set of fresh code words, such as dopamine, serotonin, anti-psychotic drugs and pharmacology.

Black patients were consistently diagnosed with more severe mental illnesses than whites subjecting them to heavier doses of drugs and longer hospital stays. In South Carolina, for example, a third of all blacks were diagnosed with schizophrenia. A figure that's 300 times higher than it is for whites. National studies indicate that this pattern of discrimination is not confined to the south. According to one survey of selected psychiatric hospitals by the National Institute of Mental Health, blacks were 2.8 times more likely than whites to be involuntarily committed to mental hospitals. Out of shame or sloppiness most states try to keep their discrimination a secret. No southern state keeps account of the number of blacks they commit to mental hospitals each year. Many of the figures in our survey had to be compiled on a hospital-by-hospital basis. Hospitals in four states Alabama, Arkansas, Kentucky, and West Virginia refused to provide any racial breakdown of their admissions. "We're never asked to break them down that way," said Janet Jenkins, Director of Admissions at Central State Hospital in Louisville, Kentucky. "We break them down by sex, but not by the race." With the number of voluntary admissions to state hospitals declining in many states the racial disparities appear to be worsening. In both Texas and North Carolina, the only two states with consistent records, the number of black patients remained relatively steady between 1975 and '85, but the number of white patients dropped by 21 percent and 53 percent in North Carolina. The primary reason why blacks are committed to mental hospitals more frequently than whites is that they are easy targets for an arbitrary commitment system. A system the US Supreme Court has condemned as "massive curtailment of liberty." A full commitment hearing is usually held before a probate judge, although Louisiana allows a local coroner to have the final say in committing people to mental hospitals. The maximum legal length of commitment ranges from 45 days in Arkansas to unlimited terms in Alabama, Mississippi, and South Carolina, which are the only three states in the nation that allow a person to be involuntarily committed and locked up for the rest of their life with no review ever. Yes. That is still in practice.

Now I'd like to examine now the labeling of mental illness, schizophrenia, and other so-called disorders. People do suffer problems in life, and do look for what is causing them. In their desperation for a solution, they are diagnosed as mentally ill by psychiatrists. If you simply take a look at psychiatry's so-called textbook on mental illness, "The Diagnostic Statistical Manual" (The DSM), you'll find that any normal behavior can be diagnosed as mental illness, and any adverse reactions to environmental influence, peer pressure and social unrest has earned a psychiatric label. If you don't wake up on time, if you sleep poorly, if you drink coffee or smoke cigarettes, or if you give up these things, if you stutter, if a child fidgets or loses things or can't wait their turn in a game, if you've ever been intoxicated, if you've had trouble with arithmetic or with grammar or with punctuation or writing expressively—all of these are now considered mental illnesses according to psychiatrists. Even teenagers who argue with their parents are, according to the DSM IV, suffering a mental disorder called "oppositional defiance disorder."

Much of the current basis of psychiatric diagnosis is rhetoric about genes and IQ creating educationally and mentally defective people. The IQ scam shows how easy it is today to diagnose anyone as schizophrenic. In the first edition of DSM in 1952 only two pages were devoted to nine different stages of schizophrenia. In 1968 the number was three pages, but the different types increased to 16. In 1980, the Insurance Guide To Schizophrenia was released in DSM III. Deregulation of the private psychiatric hospital industry began and with it, insurance companies required a formalized guide to what illnesses could be claimed against. The third edition dedicated six pages, while its revised edition in 1987 11 pages to schizophrenia. As to the point that genetic link to so-called schizophrenia was introduced with psychiatrists involved in the Germany Eugenics Movement cited as experts. In fact one of the psychiatrists cited, Carl Schneider, was a key player in the men behind Hitler and was instrumental in planning and experimenting on mental patients with drugs and then exterminating them under Nazi Operation T4. Schneider committed suicide before he could be tried at Nuremberg War Crimes Trials. This didn't stop the American Psychiatric Association from quoting his works in this prestigious diagnostic manual where terms like "familial pattern" were introduced, and we saw that biological relatives were at risk of catching this "disorder."

As schizophrenia became the cash cow for psychiatrists, the

DSM IV was released last year with 24 pages devoted to schizophrenia. Statistics studies show that psychiatrists diagnose African American males as having schizophrenia up to 1,500 percent more than they do whites. One study carried out in both 1984 and 1990 in Tennessee found that although African Americans represented only 16 percent of the Tennessee population, 48 percent of the almost 3,000 involuntary committed patients and 37 percent of the 2,100 outpatients were African American for the primary diagnosis of schizophrenia. Since 1963 the number of psychologists in schools has increased seven fold from 3,000 to 22,000. Simultaneously, SAT scores for math and verbal have plummeted. The suicidal rate among African American males between the ages of 15 and 19 has increased 125 percent since 1965. African Americans special education statistics—also a disproportionate amount of black school children are routed into special education programs compared with white school children.

Let me give you that number again. Listen carefully. Four of the five million special education students in our schools have no mental or physical disabilities. Then my question is, why would they be there?

In 1930, 80 percent of blacks over age 14 could read. In 1990 56 percent of blacks over age 14 could read. This frightening increase in illiteracy may explain why the enrollment and appropriations for both these remedial programs have ballooned, but the number of students in public schools has shrunk by several millions since the crowd of baby boomer years of the 1960s and '70s. Last year 11 million of the nation's 42 million public school students were doing primary lessons outside regular classrooms in one of these programs. A glance at expenditures for 570,000 Oklahoma public school students shows how impoverishing these programs can be. Oklahoma's total education budget was $1.7

billion; per capita funding for regular students in a standard curriculum, $22,200 per 65,000 students; and $4,000 for special education students. A major difference between American straight A private schools and her straight F public schools is that most private schools never stop teaching beginners to sound each syllable whereas most public schools started teaching or trying to teach children to sight whole words. In the US 26 percent of public school's students are in special classes. In other countries, it's one percent. Understandably many informed black parents fight to keep their children out of these classes, but sadly over half of the five million black public school students are in one of these two dead end programs.

Black patients were consistently diagnosed with more severe mental illnesses than whites subjecting them to heavier doses of drugs and longer hospital stays. In South Carolina, for example, a third of all blacks were diagnosed with schizophrenia. A figure that's 300 times higher than it is for whites. National studies indicate that this pattern of discrimination is not confined to the south. According to one survey of selected psychiatric hospitals by the National Institute of Mental Health, blacks were 2.8 times more likely than whites to be involuntarily committed to mental hospitals. Out of shame or sloppiness most states try to keep their discrimination a secret. No southern state keeps account of the number of blacks they commit to mental hospitals each year. Many of the figures in our survey had to be compiled on a hospital-by-hospital basis. Hospitals in four states Alabama, Arkansas, Kentucky, and West Virginia refused to provide any racial breakdown of their admissions. "We're never asked to break them down that way," said Janet Jenkins, Director of Admissions at Central State Hospital in Louisville, Kentucky. "We break them down by sex, but not by the race." With the number of voluntary admis-

sions to state hospitals declining in many states the racial disparities appear to be worsening. In both Texas and North Carolina,
the only two states with consistent records, the number of black
patients remained relatively steady between 1975 and '85, but the
number of white patients dropped by 21 percent and 53 percent
in North Carolina. The primary reason why blacks are committed
to mental hospitals more frequently than whites is that they are
easy targets for an arbitrary commitment system. A system the
US Supreme Court has condemned as "massive curtailment of
liberty." A full commitment hearing is usually held before a probate judge, although Louisiana allows a local coroner to have the
final say in committing people to mental hospitals. The maximum
legal length of commitment ranges from 45 days in Arkansas to
unlimited terms in Alabama, Mississippi, and South Carolina,
which are the only three states in the nation that allow a person to
be involuntarily committed and locked up for the rest of their life
with no review ever. Yes. That is still in practice.

Perhaps the best example of the change that has been taking
place in the complexion of the juvenile custody population can be
seen in the nation's response to youths involved with drugs.
Analysis shows that though murder and robbery make for bigger
headlines, drug crimes are responsible for vastly higher numbers
of juvenile arrests and incarcerations. In just one 15 year period
the per capita arrest rate for black juveniles has increased tremen-
dously and the total number of white juveniles brought into court
on drug charges is now substantially behind that of blacks, even
though blacks only make up 12 percent of the population. The
disparity is even greater for violent crimes. In one year, 32,200
more white juveniles than blacks were arrested for crimes such as
murder, forcible rape, robbery, assault and aggravated assault.
Despite that difference, 300 more blacks than whites were placed

into custody, and 2,100 more blacks than whites were transferred out of juvenile court so they could be tried in more punitive adult courts. Again, racism. Listen carefully, so you understand the meaning of this. You had 32,200 more white juveniles than blacks arrested for crimes of rape, murder, robbery, and aggravated assault. Despite that there were 300 more blacks than whites placed into custody and 2,100 more blacks than whites were transferred out of juvenile court into adult court. Across the nation this disparity is played out in almost every category of offense.

Now here's a question for you. When was the last time you heard about black women being raped? When was the last time you heard about black families being victimized and robbed? We had a white woman jogger in New York that was raped and brutalized. It was a terrible offense. That made news for weeks. I decided to do a little homework. During that same identical period of time that she was making headlines daily, more than 300 black women and Latino women had been raped and brutalized. Not one single mention in the media of any of them. Who then do we value more? Who's life do we feel is more sacred? I think the media speaks for a lot of people, and yet no one in the media writing the story would present themselves as racist. Goodwin joined as a Clinical Associate in 1965. Between 1981 and '88 Goodwin was the Director of the National Institutes of Mental Health Intramural Research Program. Listen carefully to what I'm going to share with you now. From 1988 to 1992 he was the Director of the now defunct Alcohol, Drug Abuse, and Mental Health Administration. His infamous February 1992 racist speech drew so much fire from black groups including the NAACP and the Black Congressional Caucus that the funding for the proposed Violence Initiative was never made. In 1992

Goodwin stepped down from Director of the one drug rehab group to become the Director of The National Institute of Mental Health. He remained the Director until his resignation in 1994. Mind you that his term was under two separate administrations. Republicans and Democrats had this man. This is what this man said in a speech given before the National Health Advisory Council on February 11, 1992. Goodwin then head of the US Department of Health and Human Services Alcohol, Drug Abuse, and Mental Health Administration likened inner city blacks to "hyper sexual monkeys." Let me give you the full context of this speech.

"If you look for example at male monkeys, especially in the wild, roughly half of them survive to adulthood. The other half die by violence. That is the natural way of life for males to knock each other off and, in fact, there are some interesting evolutionary implications of that because the same hyper aggression monkeys who kill each other are also hypersexual. So they copulate more and therefore they reproduce more to offset the fact that half of them are dying. Now one could say that if some of the loss of the social structure in the society, and particularly within the high impact inner city areas, has removed some of the civilized evolutionary things that we have built up and that maybe it isn't just the careless use of the word when people call certain areas of certain cities 'jungles.' That we may have gone back to what might be more natural without all the social controls that we have imposed upon ourselves as a civilization over thousands of years in our own evolution."

During the same speech, Goodwin revealed plans for a national violence initiative. The initiative involved principally a biomedical approach that would use 100,000 inner city children, mainly blacks and minorities, to focus mainly on brain neurotransmitter chemicals such as serotonin and their alleged role in violence. Researchers planned on using genetic and biochemical markers to "identify" potentially violent minority children as young as five years old for biological and behavioral "interventions," including drug therapy and possibly psychosurgery—all supposedly aimed at preventing violence later in adulthood. According to Goodwin, the Violence Initiative was scheduled to be the number one funded priority of the National Institutes of Mental Health. Subsequent to his February 1992 speech, public outcry prevented the initiative from being funded, but it had been up for funding. This comes from the *Science Magazine*, September 11, 1992, page 1474. "Her concerns haven't stopped Sullivan who insists there are 'no plans whatsoever to scrap the initiative even as he concedes he hasn't done a very good public relations job selling it.'" Well the idea was that if you wanted to launch a program make sure you have a good PR campaign around it. So what it came down to was this. They believed, and he specifically believed, that black children were the same as monkeys—uncontrollable sexual urges and violent. Their worth to society was their capacity to copulate and to kill. We had better protect society as a whole by identifying these children young in life, and that there were biomarkers that could determine a person's capacity for sexual violence and any other violence. That's why it was called the Violence Initiative. The Black Caucus and the NAACP were right in challenging the racist comments, but they would have supported it had it not been for his use of the terms. If it had been just "we believe we have a capacity to do gene testing to determine high rates of violence and prevent those," they would have passed. That's the unfortunate part. That the only way someone will stop is because they went so far over the top, but what if they hadn't have made those statements? Right now all across America millions upon millions of black youth would be given tranquilizers because of their biochemical potential for causing violence, and that would have been in a file. Those files would have been in registries in every insurance company, in every employment agency, in every high school and college. They would have the knowledge that, gee whiz, we have a kid here who's taking drugs because he is a sex violator and a criminal violator POTEN-TIALLY. The only way he's not creating the crime is because he's on a drug. Who's going to hire that person? Who's going to want to give him a mortgage? Who's going to want to have a relationship with that person? Yet it was just a five-year-old kid. Did they want to do this in the suburbs? No. Did they want to take 100,000 children five years old from executives within the United States and do it? That wouldn't be tolerated. Isn't it interesting what we will not tolerate among ourselves and we're only too happy to see it happen in other groups? So that's just to give you an idea of what's going on.

And also we have the medical evaluation field. Now this is another way they play this game. They look at the medical causes to psychiatric symptoms. Nearly two out of every five patients, that's 39 percent, had an active important physical disease. The mental health system had failed to detect these diseases in nearly half of the affected patients. Of all the patients examined, one in six, that's ONE IN SIX had a physical disease that was related to their mental disorder. It was either causing or exacerbating this disorder. The mental health system had failed to detect one in six physical diseases that were causing the patient's mental disorder. The mental health system had failed to detect more than half of the physical diseases that were exacerbating the patient's mental disorder. These are just some of the cases from different areas. What they were doing is, if you went in to a mental hospital with a mental disease and if you were black, whatever physical conditions you had were considered immaterial. They just weren't treated or minimally so because anything you would have said—if you said, "My back hurts"—they would have said well that's just part of your delusional psychosis. If you said, "I'm in terrible pain," they would have said "delusional psychosis." If you would have said, "I've got arthritis"—delusional psychosis. But later, when people did examine them, they found they had real physical problems that had not been treated. There is an article that was written called Psychological Symptoms of Physical Origin by Richard Hall and Michael Pompkin.

"One of the most difficult problems encountered by the practicing physician is that of distinguishing emotional from organic symptoms. Organically based symptoms that mimics psychiatric disorders are numerous and many diseases produce them. In women, endocrine and metabolic disorders are the most frequent causes of psychiatric symptoms. Early identification and appropriate treatment can avert many emotional, physical, and even legal problems for our patients. Any condition that disrupts the brain or alters its subtle balance of stimulation and inhibition can produce psychiatric symptoms. Often these symptoms are the first and only signs of an underlying physical disorder."

What this means in lay language is this: We can have a person going to a doctor and suggesting they have a physical symptom and that it's causing such physical problems that it's manifesting in some alteration of their emotions. If the doctor doesn't recognize that, then they'll classify the person as mentally disturbed, but without trying to fix the physical condition that may have caused the emotions. I know people who have been diagnosed, put into mental institutions, given electro convulsive therapy for depression. When I worked with them, I found out they merely had an under-active thyroid. Corrected the thyroid; the person is normal. They never had depression. Hence they were maltreated, mistreated, misdiagnosed. Because they were black and they were poor, they had virtually no recourse within the current system. No lawyer wanted to take on their case and no one wanted to hear their problem.

When all you have is a hammer, everything looks like a nail. When all you have to treat illness are pharmaceutical drugs, then you look for symptom clusters of an illness in order to use these drugs. Vitamin and mineral deficiencies, hypoglycemia, hormone imbalance, and organ pathology can all mimic depression. Allopathic medicine is not geared toward treating nutritional imbalance and instead looks at the resulting symptoms these imbalances create. Then it tries to suppress these symptoms with drugs.

The mind-body split has never been greater than in today's medicine. Medicine itself is split into so many specialties, each one trying to maintain its status and mystique. That means the individual is split as well. There is no one in charge of the whole person. So, when an Internist fails to "cure" a patient with fatigue, body rash, and itching, who also has anger and irritability, instead of recognizing a "toxic liver," the doctor sends his failure to a psychiatrist, saying that the patient's symptoms are "all in his head." Menopausal women who go through hormonal shifts are given synthetic hormones and antidepressant medication to treat a normal life change. Women with premenstrual tension are treated with Serafem, which looks like a new drug but it's just Prozac with a new name. Kids who can't stand being confined in a classroom after exploring the whole world via TV or the internet, are "calmed down" with Ritalin.

We continue to treat normal life events with drugs and it appears as if there is an overabundance of drugs just waiting to be slotted into people's lives. Insurance companies and HMOs are only too willing to promote drug therapy. It's far less expensive and far less time-consuming for a doctor to identify a few key symptoms and prescribe a drug. Everybody has stress, everybody is burdened with worry. These are normal aspects of everyday living. But when these normal individuals are constantly bombarded with advertising for mood-altering medications and told they have the right to permanent happiness, then their emotions have become pathologized. They have gone through a process where the disease has been created, in their perception of themselves, and the cure is immediately offered. And they go to their doctor and ask for the cure.

The elderly are prescribed a vast amount of drugs and are now being treated with electroshock when the drugs fail. Politicians say they are very concerned that the elderly can't afford their drugs. Instead of arguing to make medicine less expensive or instead of finding less expensive medicine or medicine that has fewer side effects, there is a debate about giving the elderly free access to drugs. It's a poor choice. This type of medical welfare is not looking after the welfare of the whole person by leaving out diet, nutrition, and lifestyle intervention in favor of drugs alone.

Where is medicine headed? The Genome Project put everyone's attention on our genetic makeup and the possibility that with genetic screening we can identify diseases and the predisposition to disease at birth. Genetic screening has taken a huge chunk out of the American research budget. The stakes are high to find the locks and the keys to the body through our genes. We often hear about the various disease genes, the breast cancer gene and even the depression gene. We create the notion of a diseased gene and offer the cure of inserting a healthy gene. Or perhaps we'll soon hear about a vaccine against depression. Replacing depression genes or using vaccines for depression may never be possible but it's just a continuation of defining depression where it does not exist and pathologizing life.

What does this mean for the average person who is on a bad diet with lots of sugar, artificial sweeteners like aspartame, packaged and processed foods with lots of additives and preservatives? Chances are your liver is toxic. Your liver is responsible for processing any chemicals that come into the body. And chances are you are feeling bloated, fatigued, constipated and irritable with a toxic liver. If you take those vague physical symptoms and obvious emotional symptoms to a doctor you will be diagnosed as anxious or depressed during a three-minute HMO appointment. You will then be given a prescription for a drug that will overload your liver even more with daily amounts of a synthetic chemical drug. And you will have side effects and feel more fatigued, bloated and irritable. But the mood-altering properties of the drug may make you feel better while the liver struggles to break down the drug.

4

SIDE EFFECTS OF DRUGS

Most people do not question the advice of their physician and take whatever drugs are prescribed for them. Other doctors offer an alternative, but their patients, believing that medicine is their only recourse or unwilling to exert the effort necessary to change poor habits, will ask, even pressure their doctors, for medication. Whatever the reason, our society is saturated with legal drug users, and this is causing us grave problems.

Study after study reveals that properly prescribed medicines are having adverse effects. The statistics for how many people are injured, hospitalized, and even dying from their medications is staggering. Yet the numbers are understated. They reflect only hospitals reporting such incidents. What is not taken into account is the amount of people suffering from such incidents at home where the vast majority of these drugs are taken. It has been estimated, in fact, that adverse incidences occur 28 times higher at home than at hospitals.

To make matters worse, improperly prescribed medications are on the rise. Giving a two-year old an antidepressant is medically unsound and scientifically unjustifiable. How in the world can you determine that a two-year-old is suffering from anxiety? You can't. The brain of that two-year old is still developing, as is the brain of a three- four- five- and six-year old. Yet the greedy manufacturers of these drugs are targeting an ever-younger market.

Has anyone asked what studies have been done on brain development in children taking these drugs for a period of years? The answer is none. Then how do you know what the consequences will be? The answer is no one does. What this means is the risk is borne purely by the patient who can become a victim and not by the physician or manufacturers.

In the current political light, it is not surprising that Eli Lilly was exempt from being sued for adding thimerisol mercury to vaccines under the Homeland Security Act. What in the world does suing a manufacturer for possible neurological effects from a vaccine additive have to do with homeland security? Nothing, but for the fact that Eli Lilly's CEO sits on an advisory board of the Homeland Security committee and has a strong political connection to George Bush Sr., who was on the board of Eli Lilly. These transactions are utterly transparent. But at the end of the day, we still have people receiving medications that should not be receiving them, and they are having adverse effects.

So whether you are getting a properly prescribed drug for a condition and having negative effects or whether an improperly prescribed one is harming you, the numbers are into the hundreds of thousands on the most conservative side, and possibly into the millions. This means, quite simply, that the number one cause of death in the United States is not from heart disease and not from stroke, but from your physician and the medications that are prescribed.

We therefore give you some idea of how dangerous the various medical procedures and medications are. We go beyond just the psychiatric ones to show you that across the board, in virtually every specialization, there is an enormous amount of unproven and dangerous medical practice occurring. Therefore *caveat emptor*, consumers beware. This is not to suggest that all medications for any condition are inappropriate. Clearly, some are essential, and lifesaving. But compared to how many are offered it is a relatively small number.

Antidepressant Drugs and Their Side Effects
Barbiturates
MAO Inhibitors
Tricyclic Antidepressants: Amytryptyline (Elavil)
SSRIs: Prozac, Paxil, Zoloft

SIDE EFFECTS OF DRUGS

Beyond the pathologizing of life itself, the most devastating side effect of antidepressant drugs is perhaps the false hope that the message of antidepressants give. They will never cure the underlying cause of depression. Yet, people take them with some notion, some belief, some misguided hope, a false hope, that drugs will indeed solve all their problems. Instead, these drugs cover up their symptoms, give people a false and synthetic sense of relief.

We also have to consider a whole generation of young people growing up on Ritalin who have had their behavior artificially modified from a very young age. They never learned how to deal with feelings of sadness, anger, joy, and accomplishment without the overlay of drugs. They have learned to equate drugs with how to cope and never learned how to be confident of their own abilities. As adults they don't know how to deal with normal feelings. They get depressed and fall right into the trap of thinking they need something to help them feel better. Prozac or Zoloft or any one of the other Prozac sisters comes across loud and clear in sexy TV ads telling them they don't have to learn how to cope, they can use a drug. Beyond what Ritalin does to kids' moods, according to the *Journal of the American Medical Association,* "Ritalin acts much like cocaine."[1]

According to the *New England Journal of Medicine,* since the mid-1990s, drug companies have tripled the amount of money they spend on advertising prescription drugs directly to consumers. The majority of the money is spent on dramatic television ads. From 1996 to 2000, spending rose from $791 million to nearly $2.5 billion. Authors of the NEJM paper admit that, "there is no solid evidence on the appropriateness of prescribing that results from consumers requesting an advertised drug."[2] The drug companies maintain that direct-to-consumer advertising is educational. But according to Dr. Sidney M. Wolfe of the Public Citizen Health Research Group in Washington, DC., the public is often misinformed about these ads. It's inevitable that patients go to their doctors demanding to become the images they see on TV by asking for a drug when they really want to be like the actor they see on the screen. Doctors are placed in a terrible bind and some spend valuable clinic time trying to talk patients out of unnecessary drugs; others write the prescription. Dr. Wolfe points out in an editorial accompanying this paper that one study found that "a substantial proportion of people mistakenly believe that the FDA reviews all ads before they are released and allows only the safest and most effective drugs to be promoted directly to the public."

According to Sarah Boseley of the *Guardian,* "Scientists are accepting large sums of money from drug companies to put their names to articles endorsing new medicines that they have not written—a growing practice that some fear is putting scientific integrity in jeopardy." She continued, "Ghostwriting has become widespread in such areas of medicine as cardiology and psychiatry, where drugs play a major role in treatment." Ms. Boseley interviewed Fuller Torrey, executive director of the Stanley Foundation Research Programmes in Bethesda, Maryland. He found that British psychiatrists were being paid around $2,000 (£1,400) a time for symposium talks, plus expenses, and Americans were paid between $3,000 and $10,000. Mr. Torrey is quoted as saying "Some of us believe that the present system is approaching a high-class form of professional prostitution."[3]

In 2000, Dr. Marcia Angell, former editor of the *New England Journal of Medicine*, wrote "Is Academic Medicine for Sale?" She said that in one paper on antidepressants, the authors' financial ties to the manufacturers—which must be declared—were so extensive that she had to run them on the website. She said, "We found very few who did not have financial ties to drug companies that make antidepressants."[4]

The World Health Organization's director of essential drugs and medicines policy, Jonathan Quick, wrote in the latest *WHO Bulletin*: "If clinical trials become a commercial venture in which self-interest overrules public interest and desire overrules science, then the social contract which allows research on human subjects in return for medical advances is broken."[3]

In general, drugs are tested on individuals who are fairly healthy and not on other medications which can interfere with findings. But when they are declared "safe" and let loose in society, they are going to be used by people on a lot of other medications with a lot of other health problems. Then science begins documenting the real effects. According to the General Accounting Office (an agency of the U.S. Government): "GAO found that of the 198 drugs approved by the FDA between 1976 and 1985 . . . 102 (or 51.5%) had serious postapproval risks . . . the serious postapproval risks [included] heart failure, myocardial infarction, anaphylaxis, respiratory depression and arrest, seizures, kidney and liver failure, severe blood disorders, birth defects and fetal toxicity, and blindness."[5]

THE HISTORY OF ANTIDEPRESSANT DRUGS AND THEIR SIDE EFFECTS

There are three main classes of antidepressant drugs: MAO inhibitors, tricyclic antidepressants, and selective serotonin reuptake inhibitors (SSRIs). The actions of all three rely on the fact that neurons depend on serotonin, a brain neurotransmitter, to convey messages through the nervous system. Research on serotonin has shown that some depressed people have low levels of serotonin in the brain. So, these drugs are given in order to enhance serotonin brain levels with the hope that this increase will alleviate depression. One of the main side effects of all the antidepressants is sexual dysfunction including impotence—both physically and psychologically. Patients don't want to have sex and if they did want to, they can't.[22, 23, 25]

MAO INHIBITORS

MAO inhibitors (monoamine oxidase inhibitors) were the first prescription antidepressants. They work by blocking an enzyme called monoamine oxidase, which acts to break down monoamines and eliminate them from the body. Powerful brain neurotransmitters like serotonin and norepinephrine are monoamines and if you turn off the enzyme that breaks them down, the result is more molecules building up. The effect can be like taking an SSRI drug, Prozac. There are about a dozen MAO inhibitors but the two most common ones still used today are Parnate (tranylcypromine sulfate) and Nardil (phenelzine sulfate).

MAO inhibitors actually work more rapidly than the tricyclic antidepressants but the side effects of MAO inhibitors have relegated them to the background of psychiatric drug intervention.

MAO Inhibitors interact with a chemical called tyramine, which must be broken down by monoamine oxidase enzymes. If you block the enzyme with a MAO inhibitor then tyramine builds up. Tyramine causes elevation of blood pressure, which could lead to stroke and/or heart attack. And the major catch is that tyramine is found in a lot of common foods such as beer, legumes (e.g., fava and soy beans), fermented soy products, cheese, fish, ginseng, meat, sauerkraut, shrimp paste, soups, and yeast extracts.

Beyond high pressures there is a long list of side effects of MAO inhibitors including dizziness, fainting, headache, tremors, muscle twitching, confusion, memory impairment, anxiety, agitation, insomnia, weakness, drowsiness, chills, blurred vision, and heart palpitations. Withdrawal from a MAO inhibitor should be done very slowly under a doctor's supervision.

TRICYCLIC ANTIDEPRESSANTS

The tricyclics inhibit the uptake of norepinephrine and serotonin and therefore have the same end result of the other two classes of antidepressants, MAO-inhibitors and SSRIs. They began to be used in psychiatry around the early 1950s. Imipramine (Tofranil) was one of the first tricyclics and is still one of the most-used medications in this group. Over the years there has been ongoing development of other tricyclics including amitriptyline (Elavil, Endep); desipramine (Norpramine, Pertofrane); nortriptyline (Pamelor and Aventyl); trimipramine (Surmontil); protriptyline (Vivactil); doxepin (Adapin, Sinequan); and Clomipramine (Anafranil).

The most difficult side effects to cope with are sedation, dry mouth, and impotence. But there are literally a hundred side effects listed in the *Physicians Desk Reference* which often cause people to curtail therapy. The side effects are worse than their depression. In the elderly, discontinuation of drug therapy often results in reoccurrence of depression.[35]

SELECTIVE SEROTONIN REUPTAKE INHIBITORS (SSRIs)

SSRIs inhibit the reuptake of serotonin allowing it to bathe brain neurons for longer periods of time. They also have a similar but lesser effect on two other brain neurotransmitters that affect mood, norepinephrine and dopamine.

Prozac was launched in 1987 and psychiatry or psychiatric patients were never the same. Prozac and its sister-medicines boost the levels of a neurotransmitter called serotonin in the brain.

Harvard Medical School psychiatrist Joseph Glenmullen, interviewed April 6, 2000 by the Associated Press, said, "We already know enough to indicate these drugs should be prescribed far more cautiously."[6] In his book *Prozac Backlash,* Dr. Glenmullen offers dozens of accounts of patients who have suffered "antidepressant backlash."[7] Side effects noted by Glenmullen include sexual dysfunction, memory loss, grotesque facial tics, anxiety and suicidal tendencies. Glenmullen feels that Prozac is toxic to the brain, as was eventually discovered about cocaine, some tranquilizers and other "mood brighteners." Glenmullen also said that "Withdrawal syndromes—which can be debilitating—are estimated to affect up to 50% of patients."

The Associated Press warns, "*Prozac Backlash* is packed with footnotes, which could indicate the debate may come down to a question of whose studies to believe." They might also add that it comes down to who funded the studies. "Glenmullen cites studies showing the Prozac class of antidepressants cause sexual dysfunction in up to 60 percent of users." But Eli Lilly, who is very angry with Dr. Glenmullen, says, "Prozac causes '20 to 30 percent max' of mild to moderate sexual dysfunction. For every footnote he cited [showing high rate of sexual dysfunction] I can show you other citations with larger numbers of patients that say just the opposite."

An Associated Press interview with Laura Young, vice president of community services for the National Mental Health Association, shows that her fears about *Prozac Backlash* changing people's minds about taking a potentially dangerous medication lie elsewhere. She says, "My fear with books like this is it scares people away from getting the really important treatment they need . . . and they may mess around with herbal alternatives."

Dr. Peter Kramer, who wrote *Listening to Prozac* just five years after Prozac hit the market was intrigued, yet skeptical of Prozac because of "its ability to alter personality." He "wondered whether the medication had ironed out too many character-giving wrinkles like overly aggressive plastic surgery." He likened Prozac to "cosmetic psycho-pharmacology." He too wondered how Prozac differs from "amphetamines or cocaine or even alcohol" both in their addictive natures and mood altering natures.[8]

Dr. Peter R. Breggin, who has been called "the Ralph Nader of Psychiatry," has written several books critical of Prozac, Ritalin, and other psychiatric drugs.[9-14] Dr. Breggin has practiced psychiatry since 1968. From the outset of his career Dr. Breggin alerted the medical profession, media, and the public "about the potential dangers of drugs, electroshock, psychosurgery, involuntary treatment, and the biological theories of psychiatry."[15] His first book in 1979, *Electroshock: Its Brain-Disabling Effects*, exposed the horror and dangers of electroshock therapy for depressed patients.[16]

For thirty years, Dr. Breggin has served as a medical expert in many civil and criminal suits including product liability suits against the manufacturers of psychiatric drugs. His work provided the scientific basis for the original combined Prozac suits and for the more recent Ritalin class action suits.[17]

The Canadian Broadcasting Corporation News and Current Affairs show did a television documentary in 2001 on the bitter controversy surrounding Dr. David Healy and The Centre for Addiction and Mental Health. The center is one of the country's top research centers and is affiliated with the University of Toronto. The university receives funding from pharmaceutical companies. The documentary said, "Dr. Healy is an expert on anti-depressant drugs such as Prozac and the center offered him a prestigious job. But then suddenly it changed its mind. The decision, the critics say, was influenced by the center's relationship with powerful drug companies."[18]

SmithKline Beecham (now GlaxoSmithKline) was sued by relatives of Donald Schell. As reported in the *Guardian*, "The court found that the company's best-selling antidepressant, an SSRI called Seroxat, had caused Schell to murder his wife, daughter and granddaughter and commit suicide."[3] The Guardian interviewed Dr. Healy who said that the company found no increased risk of suicide for depressed people on Seroxat. "But the raw data probably does not support that. Some of the placebo suicides took place while patients were withdrawing from an older drug. When the figures are readjusted without these, they show there is substantially increased risk of suicide on Seroxat." The family was awarded $8 million for their loss.[19]

THE DARK SIDE OF ANTIDEPRESSANTS

What follows is a list of side effects compiled from peer-reviewed journals. This is a sampling and not a definitive list.

Amitriptyline, Mianserin, and Unilateral ECT—side effects in patients with refractory depression[60]

Antidepressant medication—sexual dysfunction[44]

Antidepressant medication—consumer information on pharmaceutical company web sites is limited and makes it difficult to compare drugs[55]

Antidepressant therapy—sexual dysfunction in patients with depressive disorders[41]

Antidepressant treatment—sexual dysfunction in patients with anxiety and mood disorders[42]

Benzodiazepines—exert an inhibitory function on the immune system[63]

Benzodiazepines—side effects on management of insomnia[64]

Benzodiazepines—abuse, addiction, tolerance, and dependence in use[65]

Benzodiazepines—shown to be addicting both in combination with other drugs and alone[66]

Benzodiazepines—long-term use leads to dependence[67]

Benzodiazepines—patterns of use, tolerance and dependence[68]

Benzodiazepines—update on precautions to prevent abuse[69]

Benzodiazepines—dihydrohonokiol (a potent anxiolytic compound) does not result in the development of benzodiazepine-like side effects such as motor dysfunction, central depression, amnesia, or physical dependence[70]

Benzodiazepines—compromises maximum therapeutic response during a course of unilateral ECT[71]

Benzodiazepines (diazepam)—short-term use leads to a brief fugue-like state with retrograde amnesia[72]

Benzodiazepines—elderly chronic users have a significantly higher risk of cognitive decline[75]

Clomipramine—substantial adverse events in the treatment of obsessive-compulsive disorder[76]

Elavil—sleepiness; Zoloft—anxiety, agitation, headache, nausea, diarrhea, and sexual dysfunction; Paxil—dry mouth and constipation[52]

Electroconvulsive therapy—plasma prolactin levels higher following bilateral and unilateral ECT, but they were much higher after the bilateral ECT[77]

Electroconvulsive therapy—significant headaches occur in up to 45% of patients receiving ECT[78]

Electroconvulsive therapy—depressive outcome and adverse effects of ECT are independent of age, although older patients have a higher risk of developing dementia.[79]

Electroconvulsive therapy—impairment of both verbal and non-verbal functions with bilateral ECT[80]

Electroconvulsive therapy—brief-pulse ECT resulted in less memory impairment than sine-wave ECT during the first hour after treatment but had similar effects on memory after the first hour[81]

Electroconvulsive therapy—memory complaints arise from ECT as distinguished from those due to depression[82]

Electroconvulsive therapy—depression and ECT independently affect memory, and recovery from depression is not a consequence of the amnestic action of the treatment[83]

Electroconvulsive therapy—retrograde amnesia follows ECT[84]

Electroconvulsive therapy—ECT induced impairments of concentration, short-term memory and learning, and treatment-resistant patients were more likely to complain of memory problems 6 months later[85]

Electroconvulsive therapy—visual memory impairment[86]

Electroconvulsive therapy—LTP (long-term potentiation)-like long-lasting synaptic changes[87]

Electroconvulsive therapy—produces postictal disorientation; interictal disorientation increased with the number of treatments[88]

Electroconvulsive therapy—elevated cortisol predicts a greater degree of ECT-induced cognitive impairment[89]

Electroconvulsive therapy—patient developed an 18–second asystole, followed by bradycardia of 40 beats per minute for 10 seconds[90]

Electroconvulsive therapy—right unilateral (RUL) ECT associated with significant anterograde memory impairment in the short term[91]

Electroconvulsive therapy—severe cognitive impairment in geriatric patients and those with a history of interictal delirium[92]

Electroconvulsive therapy—adverse effects on memory and cognition in dementia patients who also suffer from depression[93]

Electroconvulsive therapy—bilateral ECT produces more profound amnestic effects than RUL ECT, particularly for memory of impersonal events[94]

Electroconvulsive therapy—speed of response was significantly greater when ECT was administered three times weekly but this schedule induced more severe memory impairment[95]

Electroconvulsive therapy—magnitude of retrograde amnesia for autobiographical events correlated with increased theta activity in left frontotemporal regions[96]

Electroconvulsive therapy—persisting memory loss for information acquired only a few days before treatment[97]

Electroconvulsive therapy—the hypothesis of less memory loss in the group receiving a weaker stimulus was not supported[98]

Electroconvulsive therapy—patients who manifest global cognitive impairment before treatment and patients who experience prolonged disorientation in the acute postictal period may be the most vulnerable to persistent retrograde amnesia for autobiographical information[99]

Electroconvulsive therapy—retrograde amnesia with ECT[100]

Electroconvulsive therapy—patients receiving bilateral ECT reported more symptoms of general difficulty remembering things, difficulty describing events before hospitalization, and difficulty remembering daily events[101]

Estrogen (premarin)—no meaningful effect on cognitive performance, dementia severity, behavior, mood and cerebral perfusion in female Alzheimer's Disease patients. Therefore, its therapeutic effectiveness is in doubt[20]

Estrone—a positive correlation between estrone and depression in elderly women[21]

Human immune system response—links to the temporal cycles of mood disorders[56]

Imipramine—dry mouth, sweating, and increased heart rate in long-term management of panic disorder with agoraphobia[25]

Immune-inflammatory alterations—dipeptidyl peptidase IV and adenosine deaminase activity decrease in depression[58]

Immune-inflammatory response—increased serum interleukin-1–receptor-antagonist concentrations in major depression[57]

Lithium carbonate—severe aggressive and explosive behavior in younger children more than older children[22]

Lithium carbonate—enuresis, fatigue, ataxia, vomiting, headache, and stomach ache in aggressive children[23]

Lithium carbonate—nausea, vomiting, and urinary frequency in hospitalized aggressive children and adolescents with conduct disorder[24]

Lorazepam—inappropriate secretion of antidiuretic hormone[73]

Older antidepressant medications—dry mouth, constipation, dizziness, blurred vision, and tremors; Zoloft—sexual problems; Paxil—sexual problems; Prozac—diarrhea, nausea, insomnia, and headache[62]

Prozac—severe hyponatremia in elderly patients[26]

Prozac—inappropriate secretion of antidiuretic hormone in elderly women[27]

Prozac—inappropriate secretion of antidiuretic hormone in elderly psychiatric inpatients[28]

Prozac—dangers of fluoxetine[29]

Prozac—interstitial pneumopathy induced[30]

Prozac—secondary hyperthyroidism[31]

Prozac—movement disorder[32]

Prozac—subhyaloid haemorrhage[33]

Prozac—induces anaesthesia of vagina and nipples[34]

Prozac—inappropriate secretion of antidiuretic hormone[35]

Prozac—tremors induced[36]

Prozac—causes inappropriate secretion of antidiuretic hormone[37]

Prozac—late-onset restlessness, tension, agitation, and sleep disturbances after long-term treatment[39]

Prozac—acute locomotor effects in young and aged Fischer rats[40]

Prozac—increases plasma concentrations in SSRI (selective serotonin reuptake inhibitors) and CNS (central nervous system) drug interactions[46]

Prozac—increases plasma concentrations in SSRI (selective serotonin reuptake inhibitors) and CNS (central nervous system) drug interactions[46]

Prozac—urinary retention in combination with risperidone[47]

Prozac—anxiety-like effects in male Sprague-Dawley rats[49]

Prozac—psychomotor agitation during pharmacotherapy[51]

Psychoneuroimmunology of depression—the potential for biobehavioral interventions to impact psychological adaptation and the course of immune-related disease[59]

Psychotropic drugs (benzodiazepines)—addiction, paradoxical aggressive reactions, and psychomotor automatism[74]

SSRI antidepressants, mirtazapine, venlafaxine XR—associated with higher rates of sexual dysfunction[61]

SSRI (selective serotonin reuptake inhibitors)—sexual dysfunction[48]

SSRI (selective serotonin reuptake inhibitors)—emotional blunting associated with SSRI-induced sexual dysfunction[43]

SSRI (selective serotonin reuptake inhibitors)—sexual dysfunction[45]

SSRI (selective serotonin reuptake inhibitors)—sexual dysfunction[50]

Tricyclic antidepressants—unacceptable side effects[53]

Tricyclic antidepressants—reoccurrence of unipolar depression in the elderly on discontinuation[54]

Dozens of research papers echo the concern about the side effects of SSRIs. The effects of a drug that inhibit potent neurotransmitters can't help but have profound effects on innumerable body functions. It's only since their release have we been able to fully document these side effects. Doctors have reported that patients taking Prozac have severe sodium loss[26], and severe fluid and electrolyte imbalances from inappropriate secretion of antidiuretic hormone (ADH) caused by Prozac.[27,28,35,37,38]

Prozac also affects different organ systems and causes interstitial lung disease[30]. There could also be a very real danger of increasing the already high incidence of hypothyroidism with the use of Prozac.[31] Yet, Prozac also causes hyperthyroidism.[31]

A bizarre complication of Prozac-induced anesthesia of vagina and nipples implies interference with female sexual hormones due to the drug.[34] And sexual dysfunction from SSRIs has led to management protocols[45,48,50] which may or may not include taking yet another drug, such as Viagra.

It appears that no part of the body is left unmolested—even eye hemorrhages have also occurred with the use of Prozac.[33]

Children and adolescents on Prozac have experienced movement disorders,[32,51] adults have experienced tremors,[36] and animal studies continue to show locomotor side effects with SSRIs.[40]

Drug interactions form another large segment of those patients adversely affected by SSRIs. When an other medication is used that has an effect on the brain or central nervous system, there can be negative side effects.[46] One particular drug combination causes urinary retention.[47] Studies are being done to add other drugs to the SSRI protocol to help reduce anxiety, a common side effect.[49] We haven't fully analyzed the side effects of SSRIs yet it is being given in combination to suppress some of these side effects, which can only lead to more and more complications. And yet another study comparing tricyclics to SSRIs says that SSRIs are very effective for treating anxiety and depression and should be used for patients who suffer from both conditions.[53]

Studying the literature surrounding SSRIs we find a flurry of research around depression and the immune system.[55–59] It appears that the field of psychoneuroimmunology is being overtaken in an attempt to find another class of drugs that will manipulate our immune systems. But what we've learned from our inventory of side effects of antidepressant medication tells us that we are flirting with danger when we make attempts to manipulate any part of our body's complex and unique chemistry.

5

ALTERNATIVE TREATMENTS FOR BODY, NUTRITION AND DIET

ONE of the surest ways of 'treating' mild to moderate depression in our society is to help people realize that their feelings of sadness or inadequacy may not be depression at all. Some of these feelings may, in fact, be side effects of advertising. Advertising makes people feel they lack something or are missing out on something, so they will buy a product to make up for that lack. But, it's more pervasive than that, it's as if television and glossy magazines broadcast a way of life that we are made to covet. Kids clamor for toys and sugar-coated cereals and adults clamor for an impossibly sugar-coated way of life. From "Happy Days" to "Friends" we are being brainwashed into believing that we need to be happy all the time.

Undiagnosing depression in the majority of people given this label is the best form of therapy. It would also get people off antidepressants and their inevitable and innumerable side effects, which have become an accepted part of drug therapy. It makes sense to avoid those drugs as much as possible. Fortunately there are many ways to deal with stress and feelings of depression naturally. Going for a long walk, deep breathing, repeating a positive affirmation, or burning incense, sage, or even tiny amounts of tobacco in the Native American tradition, all lend an air of ritual to your life and allow you time to dialogue with your inner self. Finding a positive connection with your inner self can help to strengthen your resolve and your confidence.

You are what you think and you are what you eat. If you eat junk food you have to put up with junk emotions. Diets loaded with sugar and white flour play havoc with your internal chemistry leading to hypoglycemia and diabetes and emotional imbalance. Processed foods are deficient in the necessary vitamin and mineral co-factors required in all the metabolic functions of the body. The liver and the nervous system depend on B vitamins and magnesium to name just two. If these nutrients are deficient, signs of anger, irritability, and anxiety are not far behind.

The research that we've accumulated on diet, nutrition, and alternative modalities for the treatment of depression is vast. It gives you many more choices and options compared to the 'elephant gun' approach of allopathic medicine, which mainly tries to manipulate your neurotransmitters. The more we learn about natural approaches with herbs and nutrients we find that they too affect neurotransmitters but in a much more subtle and balanced way.

Beyond nutrition, supplements, and herbs the following modalities such as electro-acupuncture, etc. etc., all of which are noninvasive and have proven to be beneficial in many research trials and have few if any side effects.

Many people when depressed feel unsure about what steps to take. When they see a doctor they are given certain drug options. But they are not told there are many natural or noninvasive treatments which don't have the negative side effects of pharmaceuticals. For example, here are 10 studies showing the benefits of acupuncture and electroacupuncture:

Chinese medicine practitioners use acupuncture and electo-acupuncture (hooking up acupuncture needles to small electrical currents for greater stimulation) for balancing the body's energy. They don't specifically treat depression but look upon depression as an imbalance. If a patient comes with a chief complaint of depression the whole person is assessed. Pulses are taken at the wrist, which indicates what meridians are out of balance; then acupuncture needles are put into specific points mapped along the body corresponding to certain lines or "meridians." The result is a shift in energy and relief of symptoms of depression. Perhaps the symptoms of depression were, just that, an energy imbalance. But in Western terms they were diagnosed as depression but responded to the Eastern "art" of medicine, acupuncture.

CHALLENGING THE OFFICIAL MODEL

When you go to a doctor with few non-specific symptoms such as fatigue, insomnia, and apathy that have begun to be of concern, you are usually given the label of depression. The doctor may ask some perfunctory questions about stress and tension in your life, to which most people can answer, "yes," and the diagnosis is made. You may be told that you should learn to relax and slow down but the easiest and most common treatment of depression is medication.

Not only are your symptoms of fatigue, insomnia, and apathy misdiagnosed but on medication those symptoms are going to be masked by chemicals that manipulate your neurotransmitters. Any symptoms you present with after introduction of these drugs will be evidence of your ongoing depression and need to increase your medication or add additional anti-depressants to the mix.

There are hundreds of diagnosable conditions that are overlooked when fatigue, insomnia, and apathy are misdiagnosed as depression. The following is only a partial list that includes many references to allergies because they produce chemical complexes that affect the brain.

Sugar intolerance causing symptoms of hypoglycemia and pre-diabetes that go undiagnosed. Gluten allergy from rye, oats, wheat, and barley causes particular chemicals to affect the brain. Some people are allergic to dairy products and the resulting intestinal flora imbalance leads to brain allergy symptoms. Similarly mold allergy from various foods including peanuts and two-day old left-overs, mold allergy from tobacco, and mold allergy from mildew in your home can all cause mental and emotional symptoms that some people misinterpret as depression. Allergy to fermented foods beverages including alcohol can cause emotional symptoms as can sensitivity to the hundreds of additives, dyes, colorings, and preservatives in our food and beverages.

Artificial hormones injected into beef and poultry can affect meat, dairy, and eggs that are produced and pass on allergenic triggers that affect the nervous system. In fact, allergy, sensitivity, or poisoning can occur from one of more of the hundreds of chemicals in our air, water or food, including fluoride, chlorine, pesticides, and herbicides, which can affect the brain. Heavy metal poisoning including: mercury, lead, arsenic all have a well-known history of causing symptoms from mental retardation to insanity.

The Physicians Desk Reference lists hundreds of prescription drugs with the side effect of emotional instability and depression. Depression is also common in the face of vitamin, mineral, amino acid and essential fatty acid deficiencies. None of these deficiencies are studied carefully in hospital settings for doctors to develop an appreciation of how important nutrients are to mental health. Even simple hormonal deficiencies such as adrenal insufficiency, thyroid hormone deficiency, DHEA deficiency along with the more common estrogen, progesterone, and testosterone deficiencies are mostly overlooked by busy doctors who still view the mind and body as separate.

There are many infectious causes of depression. We know that viral hepatitis can cause mental instability, the same can be said for chronic fungal, (Candida) and parasitic, infections. Inflammatory bowel disease, whether caused by infection or food allergy, causes punctures in the lining of the intestines, which allow incompletely broken down food molecules to enter the blood and act as allergens.

We also want to show you that misdiagnosis is very common in everyday medical practice when the medical model, based on scientific proof, is applied to many other diseases.

During the past century, a medical establishment has evolved that has made itself the exclusive provider of so-called scientific, evidence-based therapies. The paradigm used by this establishment is what we call the orthodox medical approach, and for the first 70 years of this century, little effort was made to challenge it. In the past 30 years, however, there has been a growing awareness of the importance of an alternative approach to medical care, one that, either on its own or as a complement to orthodox medicine, emphasizes nontoxic and noninvasive treatments, and prevention

Unfortunately, this new perspective has been fought vigorously. We've been told that it's only the treatments of orthodox medicine that have passed careful scientific scrutiny involving double-blind placebo-controlled studies. Concomitantly, we've been told that alternative or complementary health care has no science to back it up, only anecdotal evidence. These two ideas have led to the widely accepted "truths" that anyone offering an alternative or complementary approach is depriving patients of the proven benefits of safe and effective care, and that people not only don't get well with alternative care, but are actually endangered by it.

By getting society to accept these precepts, orthodox medicine has maneuvered itself into being the sole provider of information about disease and its treatment and has taken charge of curricula, accreditation, and insurance coverage in the health care arena. All 50 states have enacted strict proscriptions at the state medical board level against using so-called unscientific medicine, meaning anything that is not, according to the orthodox consensus, common-use medicine. Hundreds of physicians have been prosecuted and punished for not confining their treatments to the accepted paradigm, some to the point of having their licenses revoked, being imprisoned, or suffering bankruptcy. And it has been of only secondary importance whether or not their patients have claimed to benefit from their treatments. The prosecutors—the state attorneys general working hand-in-hand with state medical boards and "anti-quackery" groups supported by pharmaceutical interests—have influenced such federal enforcement agencies as the FDA, the USDA, and the Justice Department. They've also influenced such bodies as the National Institutes of Health as to which modalities receive funding and get incorporated into the standard medical model, thus perpetuating the status quo.

It is the purpose of this review to question the status quo. Specifically, we'll be looking at a variety of areas—cancer, heart disease, mental illness, obstetrics and gynecology, psychiatry, etc.—and asking some basic questions:

1. Are the orthodox medical modalities safe and effective, i.e., have they been proven so by qualified science?

2. If they have not been proven safe and effective, then what are the risk/benefit ratios of using these modalities?

3. What are the costs, in terms of morbidity and mortality, as well as dollars and cents, of using these modalities, both to the individual and to society as a whole?

After a careful consideration of the answers, we can determine how much of the existing mainstream medical model should be supported and how much should be rejected and replaced with new approaches.

It is vital to note that all the studies referred to here are from mainstream medicine's own respected journals, such as the *Journal of the American Medical Association*, the *New England Journal of Medicine*, and *The Lancet*. Thus this book's criticism of the various therapies comes not from the "alternative" world but from the very heart of orthodox medicine itself and from researchers using the gold standard of rigorously set-up controlled studies. So there is nothing subjective or political about the conclusions. Also, I should mention that this work was done over a period of eight years, during which time more than 10,000 studies were analyzed. The studies contained herein are just samples; many more could have been included but were not because of space considerations.

With more than 5,000 physicians questioned, it is apparent that the vast majority of medical procedures are done with the belief that they are safe and effective, rather than with proof that they are. Even after procedures and medications have been shown (a) not only not to work, but (b) to cause injury and death at a statistically significant level, they continue to gain in popularity and use. This is one of the reasons we have not had greater gains in combating the major diseases in recent decades. And it is also why there is an urgent need for physicians, legislators, journalists, funding agencies, curriculum developers, insurance companies, and peer review systems to take note of the substantial gaps in primary chronic care and find better approaches.

The facts here speak for themselves. We are a society that states that we live by the gold standard of scientific research, but this book shows that statement to be at odds with reality. It shows that we are routinely causing iatrogenic conditions and unnecessary suffering, not to mention wasting vast sums of money through a systemic negligence of the facts. This situation must be challenged and remedied. So look at the facts we present herein. It may be tedious but at the end of the day the facts must carry the day.

But why are we challenging the standard medical model? Because patients with depression and anxiety are not aware of the consequences of an incorrect diagnosis. We will show it can be lethal. By presenting just a random review of the application of this model to other diseases the reader can see that there is a larger pattern of misdiagnosis that carries over to the diagnosis of depression and anxiety. And the problem is in the general model. You don't believe us? The BMJ published an article in 2000 that reviewed the incidence and nature of medical errors in U.S. hospitals and found that 48,000–98,000 were killed each year and and additional 1,000,000 were injured. When determined the incidence of adverse drug reactions by reviewing patients' medical charts and by conducting interviews with physicians, they found that 6.5% of hospitalized patients developed an adverse drug reaction, and another 5.5% developed a potential adverse drug reaction; these events were found to be caused by errors in 28% of cases. Another study calculated that every year treatment-related complications result in 116 million additional physicians visits, 76 million prescriptions, 17 million emergency department visits, 8 million hospital admissions, 3 million long-term care facility admissions, and 200,000 additional deaths, for a cost of $76.6 billion. These data, however, significantly underestimate the real extent of the problem, since they only refer to hospital patients, and are not inclusive of errors occurring in nursing homes and other health care settings.[1a] Another article in the BMJ during the same year reported on some of the data that emerged from the results of two studies conducted by the Institute of Medicine showing that, every year, approximately 100,000 patients die needlessly in the hospital as a result of errors in medical management, and many more are injured. And the article adds that 50%-96% of adverse events are not reported. It concludes that preventable deaths from errors in medical management have reached endemic proportions, and that the extent of the injury is largely underestimated.[2a]

The reason for many of the iatrogenic mistakes is that the research the standard model claims is "scientific" is not so at all. In 1994 an article published in the BMJ questioned the integrity of the medical research community responsible for the production and publication of scientific articles in which statistical analysis are often used wrongly, studies are poorly designed, results are misinterpreted and selectively reported, and unjustified conclusions are drawn. It emphasized that all of the above phenomena are frequently found in the medical literature and are due to physicians' pressure to publish in order to advance in their career. The consequences of the poor quality of research can be devastating since patient treatment is often based on trial results which can be statistically manipulated to prove the safety and effectiveness of a specific treatment. The article concluded that "there may be greater danger to the public welfare from statistical dishonesty than from almost any other form of dishonesty."[3a] Another indication of the unscientific protocols of mainstream research were explained in BMJ in 1999 when an article highlighted that trials supported by pharmaceutical companies are significantly more likely to report favorable outcomes associated with use of the sponsored drug, compared to non-sponsored trials.[4a] Besides the unscientific milieu which produces flawed treatments, iatrogenic problems arise because the unproven treatments, usually pharmaceutical, enter the doctors' offices through dubious conflicts of interest. In 2000 JAMA published a study that indicated that pharmaceutical companies significantly influence physicians' professional behavior through gifts, free meals, sponsored travels, teachings and symposia.

It found that every year the pharmaceutical industry spends more than 12 billion dollars to push drugs, and invests an estimated $8,000 to $13,000 on each U.S. physician. While 85% of medical students judge as unethical for politicians to accept gifts, only 46% of them believe it is improper to accept a gift of similar value themselves from a pharmaceutical company. The article concluded that "the interaction between physicians and the drug-industry could have crucial consequences if it can be demonstrated that such relationship results in changes in prescribing practices toward drugs that are more expensive or that are associated with negative health outcomes."[5a] The BMJ is not waiting for such a "demonstration" because it published an article in 1999 that referred to studies on contacts between doctors and drug companies' sales representatives that demonstrated that the more doctors rely on information from drug company representatives, the less rational their prescribing is. It therefore recommended there are indeed strong reasons for physicians not seeing representatives.[6a] But the drug companies' influence is not only corrupting the studies that are being published in supposedly "scientific" journals. Now the journals themselves are becoming compromised as shown in a study that alleges that medical organizations are increasingly becoming dependent on the drug industry for their income which can pose a threat to their objectivity. The study evaluated the profits of the clinical journals of several leading medical organizations, including the *Journal of the American Medical Association*, the *New England Journal of Medicine*, the *Journal of the American College of Cardiology*, *Annals of Internal Medicine*, *Clinical Infectious Diseases*, and others. Drug advertisement contributed from $715,000 to $18 million of revenue, a sum that, according to the study, could place the organization in a position of dependency. The study also revealed that more than 10% of the income of 5 medical organizations came from drug advertisements published in a single journal, while 4 organizations profited as much or more from drug advertisement as from members.[7a]

Meanwhile, as the hoax of the "scientific" foundations for modern medicine increasingly unravels, the disastrous consequences from iatrogenic errors begin to produce studies that make obvious the need for patients in chronic care to be extremely cautious in listening to their physicians, even during the established procedures for diagnosis. An article in 1996 emphasized that 60% of routine tests conducted on patients in preparation of their surgery were unnecessary and added an extra $18 billion to the annual health care bill. In addition, unnecessary tests caused harm resulting from complications associated with the testing procedure, or with the unnecessary treatment of patients who received a false positive test result.[8a] A 1993 study reviewed all relevant articles published in English, French and Spanish from 1966 to 1992, and concluded that the costs of routine chest x-rays are so high, and the benefits so small, that its use is no longer justified in patients who have received a careful anamnesis and clinical evaluation.[9a] In the particular case of fecal occult blood screening for colorectal neoplasia, Ahlquist et al. found, in a study conducted on over 13,000 individuals, that two of the most widely used tests for the detection of colorectal cancer, the Hemoocult and Hemoquant tests, which are designed to spot the presence of occult blood in the stools, missed approximately 70% of cancers that were later diagnosed by other methods, and 90% of polyps (pre-cancerous conditions) 1 cm. or more in size.[10a]

Once the patient surmounts the hurdles blocking accurate diagnosis, there are the dangers of predominant treatments which have not been properly studied. Use of nonsteroidal anti-inflammatory drugs (NSAIDS) are now an important cause of hospitalization for congestive heart failure in individuals with or without a history of heart disease. Heart failure affects approximately 4.6 million Americans and this condition represents the most common hospital discharge diagnosis among patients older than 65 years. If this association is casual, as the dose-response relation suggests, cardiovascular morbidity due to NSAIDs would surpass gastro-intestinal NSAID-related morbidity, which alone is responsible for a minimum of 105,000 hospitalizations and 16,500 deaths occurring each year in the U.S. The economic and health consequences of these findings are staggering.[11a] A study presented at the American College of Cardiology's 49th annual scientific meeting held in California showed that hormone replacement therapy has no beneficial effects on the cardiovascular system. The study was conducted on 309 post-menopausal women with coronary heart disease who were randomly assigned to receive one of three treatments: estrogen, estrogen plus progestin, or placebo. No differences in disease progression were observed between the three groups, suggesting that neither estrogen alone nor estrogen combined with a progestin, offer protection to women from heart disease.[12a] A second study compared the effects of hormone replacement therapy, placebo, no therapy, or vitamins on the incidence of cardiovascular diseases. The results of the analysis indicated that women who took hormones had a 40% increased risk of cardiovascular events other than pulmonary embolism and deep vein thrombosis, and a 64% increased risk of cardiovascular events including venous thrombembolism, compared to women who did not take hormones. These results are in contrast with the commonly held assumption that hormone replacement therapy prevents cardiovascular diseases. Yet hormone replacement therapy is widely prescribed for American women.[13a] Many American women are routinely advised to take birth control pills but did their doctor tell them of a recent study, conducted on 46,000 women followed-up for 25 years, that demonstrated that users of oral contraceptives have a 2.5 increased risk of death from cancer of the uterine cervix, a twofold increased risk of death from cerebrovascular diseases, and a 5–fold increased risk of death from liver cancer compared to nonusers? The study also found that the adverse effects on mortality persisted for 10 years after interruption of oral contraceptive intake and ceased afterwards.[14a] Yet the common assumption is use of oral contraceptives is associated with an 80% decreased risk of death from ovarian cancer. Another study showed that women of childbearing age using combined oral contraceptives had an almost 10–fold higher risk of dying from pulmonary embolism, compared to nonusers. The finding of a substantial increased risk of this fatal complication in users of oral contraceptives is especially important when considering that these deaths occur in healthy young women who would have otherwise had a long life expectancy ahead of them.[15a] Now women who want to have children suffer the same iatrogenic effects as those avoiding childbirth—if they listen to their doctor. Almost 10 years ago a study conducted on a sample population of 3,837 women who received fertility drugs found that use of these drugs is associated with a 2.4–fold increased risk of invasive or borderline ovarian cancer, compared to non-use.[16a] Once the pregnant American woman is giving birth, another problem surfaces: in the U.S., almost 1 out of 4 deliveries is performed by Cesarean section. These rates are among the highest recorded in the developed countries. From 1970 to 1993, overall rates of primary Cesarean sections increased 4–fold, from 5.5% to 22.8%. Deliveries by Cesarean section carry a significantly higher risk of complications for both the mother and the newborn.[17a] Another study done about the same time highlighted how decisions concerning the need for Cesarean delivery seem to be influenced more by social, economic, and physicians' personal reasons than by medical factors. This is well illustrated by the fact that those women who are at highest risk of pregnancy complications and who would benefit the most from a Cesarean section are the least likely to receive it. On the other hand, indications such as previous Cesarean, slow or difficult labor or delivery, presentation of the rear of the baby at the uterine cervix and fetal distress, are the main reasons for performing a C-section, even though these conditions have been least clearly associated with benefits for the fetus and the mother.[18a]

Now let's look at prevalent health problems and note the side effects of established treatments supposedly backed up by scientific standards. A recent study showed that asthma patients receiving ipratropium bromide and theophylline have a 80% and 3–fold increased risk of death from respiratory causes, respectively, compared to those taking salmeterol. All three drugs are regularly used for patients with asthma of increasing severity.[19a] And an earlier study showed that the trend of prescribing corticosteroids as anti-inflammatory drugs for adult asthma to a growing number of patients, in larger doses and for longer periods of time, has been associated with an increased rate of potentially serious systemic adverse reactions such as adrenal suppression, osteoporosis, cataract, stunted growth in children, altered metabolism, and behavioral abnormalities.[20a] Reviewing the studies on treatments for cancer we find the same failures of modern claims. A study in 1997 showed that U.S. cancer mortality rates in 1994 were 6% higher than in 1970. Cancer mortality rates increased steadily for nearly two decades, reached a plateau, and then decreased by 1% from 1991 to 1994. The authors of the study say this decrease can be attributed to reduction in cigarette smoking and to early detection, but not to the effects of new treatments which have been largely disappointing. The authors conclude, "35 years of intense effort focused largely on improving treatment must be judged a qualified failure," and argue that progress can occur only through a national commitment to prevention through reallocation of funding and shift of research focus.[21a] Frezza et al. reviewed all cases of gallbladder cancer treated at Howard University during the past 28 years, plus the literature published on the subject during the last 20 years to determine the efficacy of non-surgical therapies in the management of gallbladder cancer. No improved survival was observed in patients treated with chemotherapy or radiotherapy.[22a] Nor on gastric cancer[23a], esophageal cancer[24a], head and neck cancer[25a], lung cancer[26a], melanoma[27a], pancreatic cancer[28a], renal cancer[29a], or uterine cancer[30a]. Moving along to diabetes we have a study that intensive treatment of type 2 diabetic patients with sulphonylureas or insulin, compared to conventional treatment (consisting of diet with the addition of pharmacological treatment if glucose levels cannot be controlled by diet alone), decreases the risk of microvascular complications (i.e. retinopathy, nephropathy and neuropathy) but has no effect in preventing macrovascular complications. Furthermore, patients in the intensive treatment group experienced significantly more hypoglycaemic episodes and weight gain compared to those in the standard treatment group. Weight gain was especially high in patients treated with insulin.[31a] Standard anti-epileptic drugs don't work either as D. Chadwick showed in his 1995 survey where a randomized trial by Temkin et al., conducted on a cohort of patients with seizure following head injury, showed that individuals taking the antiepileptic drug phenytoin experienced more seizures than those receiving placebo. As the author concludes, "None of the available clinical trials comparing early treatment with deferred treatment seemed to show any great benefit to longer term outcomes." These data cast serious doubts on the value of early treatment for epilepsy.[32a]. Finally be forewarned of the dangers of a stay in a hospital. In 2000 an article reported that every year in the U.S., approximately 2,000,000 patients develop hospital-acquired infections and 88,000 die from them. The cost of hospital-acquired infections has been estimated at $4.6-billion. These estimates are conservative, because they do not take into account nosocomial infections occurring in patients in nursing homes, outpatient clinics, dialysis centers and other health care centers.[33a]

6

HOLISTIC PROTOCOLS

Virginia Wolf, Ernest Hemingway, Michelangelo Buonarroti, Gustav Mahler. What did they have in common, other than greatness in their talents? They all suffered from what author Andrew Solomon very appropriately calls "The Noon-Day Demon": depression.

Dr. Jay Lombard, Board Certified Neurologist and former Chief of Neurology at Westchester Square Medical Center, author of "The Brain Wellness Plan", puts depression at the top of the list of modern epidemics. According to Dr. Lombard, 20% of adults in the U.S. experience one or more depressive episodes, while 5% receive a diagnosis of clinical depression. Of the latter group, 15% of the cases end in suicide.

An especially alarming trend is reflected by the increase in the incidence of depression among teens and young adults, and even children. It is estimated that at least 5% of American teenagers currently suffer from depression severe enough to warrant medical treatment, but these numbers may not reflect a much more alarming reality.

It is no surprise, given these statistics, that pharmaceutical companies are so eager to fund research aimed at finding effective relief for this life threatening condition. And yet, current drug treatment seems to fall short of expectations. It works sometimes, for some people, but for many it becomes a frustrating juggling act from one drug to another, waiting for an elusive relief that never seems to come, or never seems to stay.

And while the initial lessening of symptoms offered by antidepressants is desirable and necessary, it carries the potential for serious, long-term, undesirable side effects such as tardive diskenesia, paranoid and psychotic reactions, and liver malfunction, among others.

Candace B. Pert, Ph.D., is mostly known for her discovery of endorphins, the opiate-like chemicals produced by the brain and nervous system. Her pioneering work has led the way into this quickly expanding field of research and has been one of the most important foundations for establishing the bio-molecular connection between brain chemistry and emotional states.

Experts may disagree on how to treat depression, but there is an almost unanimous consent among them that depression is caused by a chemical imbalance in the flow of neurotransmitters that bathe our brains at any given moment,—too much of one or not enough of another. All it takes is a re-balancing act, research seems to promise. The task of the health care practitioner, according to this approach, lies in figuring out which chemical or chemicals are out of balance and to provide the patient with a drug that corrects the problem. If it sounds too simple to be true, it probably is. And it's the best current psychiatry has to offer.

What we did in our study is to challenge the axiom that the patient's brain chemistry is inherently faulty and therefore in need of permanent outside intervention. In other words, we changed the therapeutic stance from one that defines the patient as a passive, helpless victim of a fateful brain dysfunction to one that puts him/her in the driver seat of this delicate and possibly life-saving "brain rescue" operation.

The results of our study, we are delighted to say, have opened a window of hope for those who suffer from this very painful, often devastating condition. Indeed, we believe that this remarkable study, unique in its parameters, offers a new foundation upon which to build the future of brain research.

What is different and unique about our study was that we didn't try to forcibly re-direct brain chemistry by supplementing the participants' diet with isolated nutrients and/or herbal supplements, nor did we require that participants stop taking the medications prescribed for their symptoms. Rather, our aim was to find out whether neurotransmitter imbalances leading to depression could be the consequence of life style choices, and not an elusive brain abnormality that can only be affected by aggressive chemical interventions.

To establish whether this was true or not, we designed a parallel study where participants were given high doses of nutrients known to positively affect brain functioning, such as St. John's Wort, PS and PC complexes, SAMe, DHA, and others. No other change was required—dietary or otherwise. The outcome of this study showed that single, isolated nutrients have little or no impact on mental outlook and overall health. Symptoms of anxiety/ depression persisted, and no major positive change was noted in this group.

Participants in the first group ranged from 20 to 78 years old. In order to be accepted in to the the study, all of the participants had to present a letter from their physician stating that they had been diagnosed with, and were in treatment for, anxiety and/or depression, primary and secondary. If they were taking nutritional supplements on their own, such as a multi-vitamin or a B-complex for instance, we asked them to suspend supplementation for the duration of the study. However, we told them to continue taking their medications as prescribed by their doctor. All medical aspects of the study were closely monitored by Martin Feldman, M.D., Board Certified Neurologist.

The need for life style modification was discussed and explained in detail to the participants, and attendance to weekly meetings was made mandatory, in order to effectively monitor the evolution of the study. All of them were asked to implement the following changes:

1. Identify and eliminate all known allergens and toxins from the diet, plus learn to purchase, prepare, and enjoy good, healthy and natural foods.
2. Self-administer a simple test in order to evaluate thyroid activity.
3. Establish, maintain, and gradually increase intake of beneficial phytochemicals from fresh vegetables and fruit juices, and/or from food concentrates.
4. Avoid watching television, except for movie classics and educational programs. We also asked that participants abstain from reading upsetting news for obvious reasons.
5. Learn stress management tools, such as relaxation, meditation, prayer, positive affirmations and positive thinking techniques, and use them daily for a minimum of an hour.
6. Engage in one hour of mild to moderate daily aerobic exercise, as well as learn basic Yoga and breathing techniques.
7. Identify and correct hormonal imbalances, especially for men and women, whose hormonal status may be one of the major underlying causes of brain imbalances (i.e., reduced testosterone, thyroid, etc.)
8. And finally, perhaps most importantly, we encouraged par-

ticipants to do whatever was necessary to boost and restore efficacious immunity. For many of them, one of the greatest discoveries was linking mercury amalgam fillings in their teeth with their mental anguish: once the mercury was removed many of the gloomy feelings seemed to disappear as well.

Once the relevance of the required change was understood, its implementation was facilitated and made possible by providing participants with simple, practical information and support at our weekly meetings. These meetings lasted two hours and provided an open forum for individuals to share their experience with one another, thereby creating an opportunity for positive reinforcement of their newly learned behaviors. We also provided individual counseling and support as needed.

After three months on this program, and without any heavy-duty nutritional or herbal intervention, 93% of participants reported markedly elevated energy level; relief of anxiety and depression symptoms; improved cognition; better sleep; improvement in digestion and elimination; better focusing ability; a sense of internal peace and confidence, as well as a significant improvement in their overall mental state.

Many felt confident enough to ask their physician to lessen or discontinue their medication and thus were able to establish and maintain a stable, drug free, comfortable lifestyle. What was especially remarkable was that, along with the subsiding of anxiety and depression symptoms, all participants across the board achieved a level of overall health they had not been able to achieve or sustain previously.

We hope that this study will serve as a template for future research, and we present it in this book as a prototype for what we consider a state of the art approach to the treatment of anxiety and depression. Ultimately, it is our hope that it may establish the foundation for a more holistic and effective approach to the treatment of mental illnesses.

FOOD SENSITIVITIES, DIET, NEUROTOXINS AND BRAIN HEALTH

Our modern diet is conveniently suited for a fast paced lifestyle—one that emphasizes productivity at the expense of quality. When we consume highly processed foods, fast foods, soft drinks, caffeinated beverages and alcohol in any form, we may temporarily experience a surge of artificial energy, and we may be misled into believing that our brain's nutritional needs have been met. However, nothing could be further from the truth. The artificial stimulation that enables us to be more productive eventually takes a heavy toll on our health, possibly establishing the groundwork for depression and/or anxiety to take hold.

Even though people have unique allergy profiles determined by the individual's unique history and set of circumstances, some popular food items and drinks seem to cause allergic reactions in most people. These items include sugar- and gluten-containing products, caffeinated and alcoholic drinks, artificial sweeteners, hydrogenated fats, cold cuts and other processed meats, food containing MSG (mono sodium glutamate) and/or other flavor enhancers, preservatives and artificial color. We asked the participants in one study to abstain from these items and to avoid nicotine in any form, as well as recreational substances, legal or illegal.

In order to establish and correct individual allergies, we then taught participants two of the simplest methods of self-assessment. The first method requires that one abstain from a suspected food item for a week, then consume a considerable amount of the same food all at once. If an unusual reaction occurs, or if there is a flare-up of symptoms that had temporarily subsided, chances are that the food is allergenic for that individual.

In the other method, the food in question is eliminated from the diet, again, for one week. On the morning of the eighth day, one's pulse should be taken upon awakening, before getting up or doing anything else. After mentally recording this initial reading, the person is instructed to swallow a small piece of the food and lay in bed for twenty minutes. The heart rate is then checked again. If a five beats-per-minute increase is noted, the food is most likely causing an allergic reaction and should be eliminated from the diet, at least temporarily.

Avoiding potentially neuro-toxic and allergy causing foods is an absolute necessity, since their metabolic by-products have the capacity to interfere with normal brain functions. Because so many staples in the standard American diet fall in this category, participants in the study were given detailed instructions on how to buy fresh, organic and non-allergenic food items. They were also given recipes and explanations on how to cook these foods and prepare delicious, wholesome, vegetarian meals with the inclusion of some fish and organic poultry, if desired.

A very strong emphasis was placed on drinking freshly extracted vegetable and fruit juices, starting with one glass a day for the first week of the study and increasing by one glass each subsequent week, until total juice intake reached two quarts per day, after which it was maintained at that level. To those participants suffering from diabetes, who could not negotiate the fructose in juices, we showed how to obtain the same beneficial effects by taking fruit and vegetable concentrates from which fructose had been removed.

These comprehensive dietary changes did bring on the results we had hoped for, namely, a gradual and steady decrease in symptoms of anxiety and depression, as we reported above, in 93% of the participants.

They also brought on several desirable side effects, such as more stable glucose blood levels; improvement in cardiovascular health; weight loss or gain reflective of improved assimilation and metabolism; pain relief for those suffering from arthritis and other chronic inflammatory conditions; not to mention better memory, clearer thinking and increased libido.

STRESS MANAGEMENT

"Man does not live by bread alone." Indeed, we are constantly taking in our environment, in the form of cosmic dust, floating micro-organisms and other microscopic particles, sounds, sights, aromas, magnetic waves, and information affecting our psyche. When we focus on something, we increase our "attentional" intake of that particular object, thereby increasing its potential impact on our psychic structure. This is how we create our mental landscape, where memory, imagination and perception join together to give us a sense of what our reality is like.

In other words, what we selectively absorb from our environment determines, to a large extent, how we feel about being in it. If we allow our ears to be flooded with news of death and destruction all day long, our brain may eventually become accustomed to high levels of neurotransmitters that spell disaster, in response to what we perceive.

This kind of habitual, negative input can affect brain chemistry and eventually aggravate symptoms of anxiety and depression. So can excessive TV watching, simply as a result of magnetic waves.

For the reasons mentioned above, the first step in establishing a successful stress management strategy was for participants to abstain from watching TV or reading newspapers.

Removing potentially distressing negative input was the first step in the stress management component of our study. We basically chose the same approach we had followed in guiding the participants through the required dietary changes: first eliminate intake of known toxins (for body and mind alike), then replace negativity with positive input.

The next step was therefore to teach participants many well-known, simple and effective self-help techniques, including Yoga and deep breathing, relaxation, meditation, visualization, positive affirmations, prayer, self-hypnosis, bio-feedback, Tai Chi and Qigong, among others. We recommended engaging in any of these activities, according to individual preferences, for at least an hour a day.

Instructions on how to safely engage in mild to moderate aerobic exercise, for at least one hour a day, was the third and final element included in the stress management part of the study. As a result of this comprehensive approach, we believe, the positive changes brought on by improved nutritional status were potentiated and reinforced, thereby creating a powerful synergistic dynamic between mind and body.

This newly found sense of well being served to increase rewarding inner feelings such as a sense of peace and self-confidence. Participants felt that what they were getting out of the study was well worth the efforts required in order to participate in it.

THYROID TEST

Symptoms of depression can be caused by a malfunctioning thyroid gland. When the thyroid is impaired in its ability to regulate metabolism, the self-renewal capacity of the body is greatly reduced. The energetic stagnation that ensues is experienced as depression, fatigue and listlessness.

Because routine blood tests are not designed to detect serious thyroid malfunctioning, depressive symptoms caused by this disorder are often overlooked and treated as primary depression, thereby addressing their real cause.

To self-assess thyroid activity we told participants to place a thermometer under the armpit upon awakening in the morning, before doing anything else and record underarm temperature for seven consecutive days.

For those participants whose body temperature upon awakening was consistently low, below 98 degrees Fahrenheit, an in-depth thyroid evaluation was recommended, in order to obtain appropriate treatment for this imbalance whenever medically indicated.

ENDOCRINE AND IMMUNE REGULATION AND ENHANCEMENT

Hormones, neurotransmitters, leukotrienes, cytokines and prostaglandins are just some of the microscopic chemical messengers that, under normal circumstances, appropriately initiate, regulate or terminate many of the biological processes in the body.

These chemicals are constantly being produced, as needed, in response to the challenges and demands of daily life. They are manufacture, stored, activated, sent, received, deciphered, translated into biological changes, and finally recycled or destroyed, at every moment of our life.

Levels of these powerful chemicals can become altered as a result of inadequate diet, unhealthy lifestyle, aging coupled with nutritional deficiencies, stressful events, medication, illness or any other unusual set of circumstances.

When this happens, the whole system of communication in the body can become imbalanced. Overregulation and/or underproduction of compensatory chemicals becomes the body's strategy, one that often becomes habitual and pathological. It is easy to understand how these imbalances can offset the delicate pattern of chemical brain regulation, precipitating mood changes towards anxiety and/or depression.

For this reason we felt it was important to obtain a baseline at the beginning of the study, whereby participants' hormonal profile was assessed and recorded. In most cases, we found sub-optimal levels of the main hormones, such as DHEA, testosterone, progesterone, estrogen and melatonin, while cortisol levels were abnormally high.

At the end of the three months, without hormonal supplementation or direct regulation by any means other than health supportive lifestyle changes, we took a second reading of the participants' hormonal status. We are happy to report that, in 90% of the cases, all the major levels of hormones had normalized, while cortisol levels had dropped. For participants in their 60s and 70s, these changes were especially remarkable, since their hormonal levels had not been that high since their youth.

We took a similar approach when it came to assessing participants' immune status. A baseline of all major immune system markers was taken at the beginning of the study, including measurements of lymphocytes, macrophages, T cells, antigens and antibodies, among others.

Again, what was found was a consistency of abnormalities,

ranging from chronic immune suppression to over-regulation. As we mentioned above, a very significant improvement in immunity was noted by all participants who had mercury amalgam fillings and had them removed. By the end of the study, 90% of participants' immune status had normalized with all immune modulators back to normal levels.

From the standpoint of psychoneuroimmunology, our study proves that mental health cannot effectively be addressed as separate from, and independent of, immune processes and overall physical health. In that sense, our study was very complex, since we eliminated the dichotomy between body and mind and worked with the organism as a unit which functions on all levels simultaneously and reflectively.

We feel we have proven that the best and safest treatment modality is established when all symptoms are addressed as pertinent to the totality of who the patient is, as opposed to treating each organ and system as a separate unit that works somewhat independently of the rest of the organism.

We believe that our approach greatly eliminates the need for specialized care of isolated systems or body parts, thereby pointing to the possibility for a non-toxic, safe and cost effective approach to mental health and disease prevention in general.

Slowly increase dosages to recommendations listed below. Build up to the full protocol recommendations over the course of one month. You may start by taking a group of suggested supplements (2 or 3 at a time) to see if you have any adverse reactions. Process of elimination for allergy response will be simpler this way.

PROTOCOL FOR ANXIETY

Chromium picolinate, 200 mcg., twice a day.

Zinc citrate, 25 mg., twice a day.

Selenium, 50 mcg, twice a day.

Vitamin B; B1, 50 mg, twice a day; B6, 50 mg, twice a day; B12, 1,000 mcg, once a day; folic acid, 1,000 mcg, once a day; pantothenic acid, 600 mg twice a day; all B vitamins should be taken with food.

Vitamin C with bioflavonoids, 5,000 to 10,000 mg a day, or to bowel tolerance.

Lead-free calcium citrate, 500 to 1,000 mg.

Magnesium citrate, 500 to 1,000 mg.

5HTP, 100 mg, at bedtime (Caution: check with your doctor before taking 5HTP if you are on any of the SSRI's anti-depressants).

L-tyrosine, 1,000 mg, twice a day on an empty stomach (Caution: do not take L-tyrosine if you are taking an MAO inhibitor drug)

Taurine, 500 mg, twice a day on an empty stomach.

EFA's, 3,000 mg a day, plus 200 mg DHA.

Melatonin, 5 mg at bedtime.

Anti-oxidant formula blend, take as directed. Commonly available at vitamin outlets.

Phosphatidylserine and phosphatidylcholine complexes, or lecithin granules. Use as directed on bottle.

Herbs that have been found helpful in reducing anxiety are: chamomile, valerian, skullcap, passionflower, California poppy, St. John's Wort, and linden flower. Use as directed on bottle.

Among the more exotic remedies, one that shows great promise is called Adapton. Adapton is a natural alternative to the drugs commonly prescribed for treatment of anxiety disorders. It comes from a species of sish, called garum, which is found exclusively off the coast of England.

Adapton's efficacy has been thoroughly tested and confirmed in several studies. It has been found that the polypeptides contained in it act as precursors to endorphins and other neurotransmitters, plus it contains an omega-3 fatty acid complex that enhances prostaglandins and prostacyclins, important chemical mediators of neurological and immune functions.

Adapton has an overall beneficial effect on mental outlook and cognitive functions. Because of its safety and efficacy, it is being prescribed more and more in Europe for treatment of anxiety disorders, childhood hyperactivity, attention deficit disorder and other learning disabilities.

PROTOCOL FOR DEPRESSION

SAMe, 400 mg, 3 to 4 times a day.

Phosphatidylserine and choline complexes, 500 mg a day.

St. John's Wort, 300 mg, 2 times a day.

Gingko Biloba, 400 mg a day.

NADH, 5 to 10 mg a day

EFA's, 3,000 mg a day plus 200 mg DHA.

Glutathione, 2,000 mg a day on an empty stomach.

NAC, 1,000 mg twice a day on an empty stomach.

Acetyl-L-carnitine, 1,000 mg, twice a day on an empty stomach.

Dl-phenylalanine, 1,000 mg in the morning and 500 mg in the early afternoon, on an empty stomach (Caution: do not take dl-phenylalanine if you suffer from panic attacks, diabetes, high blood pressure or PKU).

L-tyorsine, 1,000 mg, 3 times a day, on an empty stomach (Caution: do not take L-tyrosine if you are takin and MAO inhibitor drug).

5HTP, 100 mg at bedtime (Caution: check with your doctor before taking 5HTP if you are on any of the SSRI's antidepressants).

Zinc citrate, 25 mg a day.

Selenium, 200 mcg a day.

B-complex, 100 (???? Mg or mcg), once a day.

Vitamin C with bioflavonoids, 5,000 to 10,000 mg a day or to bowel tolerance.

Vitamin E complex, 800 units a day.

Antioxidant formula, take as directed on the bottle.

Melatonin, 5 mg at bedtime.

Herbs and other remedies that may help relieve symptoms of depression: green tea, green tea extract, licorice, astragalus, ginseng, ginger, lemon balm, peppermint teas.

7

88 WAYS TO SUPERCHARGE YOUR IMMUNE SYSTEM

1. Your immune system protects you from disease
The immune system consists of various cells divided into two key groups: B-cells and T-cells. B-cells are responsible for the formation of antibodies that defend against pathogenic attack, and T-cells are responsible for cell-mediated immunity and production of chemicals and molecules that kill invading microorganisms. The immune system is also composed of the skin and various mucous membranes that, if damaged, can allow invasion. [Hunter, J.O. Food allergy—or enterometabolic disorder? *Lancet* 1991 Aug 24; 338(8765):495–6]

2. Keep your stress level low
Chronic stress can severely impact immune system function. Acute stress can increase immune response. [Hucklebridge, F., Lambert, S., Clow, A., Warburton, D.M., Evans, P.D. Sherwood, N. Modulation of secretory immunoglobulin A in saliva; response to manipulation of mood. *Biol. Psychol.* 2000 May; 53(1): 25–35]

3. Take melatonin to enhance your immune system
Melatonin boosts production of T-helper cells, which identify

cancer cells, viruses, fungi and bacteria in the body. Melatonin also enhances production of T-helper cells, gamma-interferon and eosinophils—substances that attack unwanted invaders. [Maestroni, G.J. The immunoneuroendocrine role of melatonin. *J. Pineal Res.* 1993 Jan; 14(1): 1–10].

4. Keep your immune system healthy
When disease-causing organisms invade our body, the immune system calls several different forms of cells into action, including neutrophils and macrophages. Sometimes, the so-called *complement system* will activate, made up of a group of proteins that target these invaders in tissues and blood. This system also promotes inflammation at the site of infection through the release of special chemicals like cytokines, interleukins and tumor necrosis factor (TNF-_). [Goldsby, R.A., Kindt, T.J., Osborne, B.A. *Kuby Immunology, Fourth Edition* 2000. New York: W.H Freeman]

5. Keep your immune system strong
MGN-3, a compound produced from certain mushrooms, enhances natural killer cell activity in cancer patients. It also produces beneficial activity against HIV, the virus that causes AIDS. [Ghoneum, M. Immunomodulatory and Anti-cancer Properties of MGN-3, a Modified Xylose from Rice Bran, in 5 Patients with Breast Cancer. American Association for Cancer Research Special Conference, November 5–8, 1995 (Abstr.)]

6. Managing your emotions can help your immune system
Studies have shown that there is a definite mind/body link in health. Brain cells can effectively "talk" to immune cells. Our state of mind has either a beneficial or detrimental effect on our immune system capability. [Pert, C. B. *Molecules of Emotion: Why You Feel the Way You Feel* 1999. New York: Simon & Schuster]

7. Avoid stress as often as possible

Studies show chronic stress deteriorates your immune system's capability to fight off disease. By contrast, avoiding stress can have a beneficial effect on your immune system. [Hucklebridge, F., Lambert, S., Clow, A., Warburton, D.M., Evans, P.D. Sherwood, N. Modulation of secretory immunoglobulin A in saliva; response to manipulation of mood. *Biol. Psychol.* 2000 May; 53(1): 25–35]

8. Avoid free radical invasion

Pro-inflammatory cytokines, beneficial proteins that make up the immune system, kill foreign cells in an oxidative burst of activity. This yields a large production of free radicals in our bodies. [Goldsby, R.A., Kindt, T.J., Osborne, B.A. *Kuby Immunology, Fourth Edition* 2000. New York: W.H. Freeman]

9. Be sure to take the right mix of vitamins

The right blend of nutrients can boost our immune system's capacity. The discovery of vitamins in the 19th century proved that nutrients play a critical role in helping keep our immune systems strong. [Beisel, W.R. Nutrition and immune function: overview. *J. Nutr.* 1996; 126(10 Suppl.): 2611S–2615S]

10. Take your supplements everyday.

Nutritional supplements contain a powerful mix of micronutrients that are known to boost metabolic processes that fight off disease. Lack of these critical nutrients can have an opposite effect, and help bring on disease. [Chandra, S., Chandra, R.K. Nutrition, immune response, and outcome. *Prog. Food Nutr. Sci.* 1986; 10(1–2): 1–65]

11. Be sure to take your vitamins

The right blend of vitamins can promote energy in cells, and protect against free radical invasion. They also help cells communicate with other cells in the body. [Chandra, R.K., McBean, L.D. Zinc and immunity. *Nutrition* 1994 Jan–Feb; 10(1): 7–80]

12. Vitamins have a wide range of benefits

Studies have shown that vitamins help us resist infection. There is a strong connection between the proper vitamin/mineral balance and immunity. [High, K.P. Micronutrient supplementation and immune function in the elderly. *Clin. Infect. Dis.* 1999; 28(4): 717–22]

13. Don't forget to take the right minerals

Minerals like copper, iron and zinc interact with other vitamins and minerals and help keep your immune system strong. Infants, young children and pregnant or nursing women are at especially high risk of zinc deficiency. [Chandra, R.K. Nutrition and immune responses. *Can. J. Physiol. Pharmacol.* 1983 Mar; 61(3): 290–4]

14. Take the right nutrients to fight off disease

Groups like atopic, formula-fed children, low-birth-weight infants, obese adolescents, malnourished hospitalized patients and the elderly have increased immune dysfunction. When supplements of the right nutrients are combined with healthy diets, immune function can improve. [Chandra, R.K. Nutrition and immunology: from the clinic to cellular biology and back again. *Proc. Nutr. Soc.* 1999 Aug; 58(3): 681–3]

15. Take the right combination of nutrients
Keeping the immune system strong and healthy will fight off infection and free radical invasion. There is no single nutrient or vitamin that can boost immunity as effectively as the right combination of all of them. [Lesourd, B.M. Nutrition and immunity in the elderly: modification of immune responses with nutritional treatments. *Am. J. Clin. Nutr.* 1997 Aug; 66(2): 478S–484S]

16. Take optimal blends of nutrients
The proper blend of vitamins and minerals can enhance immunity, and fight off foreign invasion, as well as the buildup of free radicals in the body. But too much of one nutrient can do just the opposite. [Delafuente, J.C. Nutrients and immune responses. *Rheum. Dis. Clin. North Am.* 1991 May; 17(2): 203–12]

17. Glutathione can boost immune function
Immune response was dramatically improved in animals fed whey protein concentrate when exposed to Salmonella, Streptococcus pneumonia and cancer-causing chemicals. [Bounous, G., Baruchel, S., Falutz, J., Gold, P. Whey proteins as a food supplement in HIV-seropositive individuals. *Clin. Invest. Med.* 1993 Jun; 16(3): 204–9.]

18. Regular exercise is good for strong immunity
Regular physical activity may boost levels of natural killer cell activity in the immune system. These killer cells attack and destroy parasitic organisms. [Shinkai, S., Konishi, M., Shephard, R.J. Aging, exercise, training, and the immune system. *Exerc. Immunol. Rev.* 1997; 3: 68–95]

19. Protect against free radicals

Oxidation can kill invading cells, but the free radicals that are produced in the process have been linked to immune system damage related to normal aging. Science has uncovered the vital role that antioxidants and other essential nutrients play in helping to ward off immune system damage. [Beisel, W.R. Nutrition and immune function: overview. *J. Nutr.* 1996; 126(10 Suppl.): 2611S2615S.]

20. Protect against free radicals

Trace elements like zinc, copper, manganese and selenium act as cofactors of antioxidant enzymes, which protect against free radical activity. Selenium, in particular, removes harmful fatty deposits called lipids from the body, protecting against a range of cancers. [Leung, F.Y. Trace elements that act as antioxidants in parenteral micronutrition. *Can. J. Nutr. Biochem.* 1998; 9(6): 304–7.]

21. Keep nutritional supplements handy

The proper combination of nutritional supplements, proteins, hormones and certain drugs can enhance the immune system. These micronutrients can protect our metabolism from the damage inflicted by free radicals. [Chandra, R.K. Nutrition and immune responses. *Can. J. Physiol. Pharmacol.* 1983 Mar; 61(3): 290–4.]

22. Don't forget essential supplements

Supplements like Echinacea purpurea and Panax ginseng significantly enhances the function of natural killer cells that make up the immune system in patients with AIDS or chronic fatigue syndrome. Extracts of echinacea and ginseng enhance cellular immune function in healthy people, as well as in those with a compromised immune system. [See D.M., Broumand, N., Sahl, L., Tilles, J.G. In vitro effects of echinacea and ginseng on natu-

ral killer and antibody-dependent cell cytotoxicity in healthy subjects and chronic fatigue syndrome or acquired immunodeficiency syndrome patients. *Immunopharmacology* Jan 1997; 35(3):
229–35.]

23. Supplements can help stave off infection

Biostim, a substance extracted from a certain bacterium, helps
fight infection, especially in those with weakened immune systems. One study showed Biostim helped severely ill patients
recover more rapidly. [Lacaille, F. Administration of RU 41740, a
preventive anti- infective immunomodulator in an acute respiratory episode. Synthesis of 3 clinical trials. *Presse Med.* 1988 Jul
27; 17(28): 1453–7 (in French).]

24. Don't forget your vitamins

Vitamins are essential for energy produced by various cells in the
body, as well as protection against oxidants. They are essential for
various cells to properly communicate with each other. Studies
have used levels of immune cells, the presence of antibodies and
the antigen-related stimulation as measures of immune activity
both in patients and in the lab. [Chandra, R.K., McBean, L.D.
Zinc and immunity. *Nutrition* 1994 Jan–Feb; 10(1): 7–80.]

25. Remember to keep nutritional supplements handy.

The supplement DHEA helps boost levels of a good protein in
your immune system. Likewise, it diminishes levels of a bad protein known as interleukin-6, a global marker of bad health. [Fer-
rucci, L., Harris, T.B., Guralnik, J.M., Tracy, R.P., Corti, M.C.,
Cohen, H.J., Penninx, B., Pahor, M., Wallace, R., Havlik, R.J.
Serum IL-6 level and the development of disability in older persons. *J. Am. Geriatr. Soc.* 1999 Jun; 47(6): 639–46; comment, *J.
Am. Geriatr. Soc.* 1999 Jun; 47(6): 755–6.]

26. Immune boosting supplements are essential

Biostim is extracted from a bacterium, and helps boost the immune system. It helps treat bronchitis, and dramatically reduces the need for antibiotics during an infection. [Viallat, J.R., Costantini, D., Boutin, C., Farisse, P. Double-blind study of an immunomodulator of bacterial origin (Biostim) in the prevention of infectious episodes in chronic bronchitis. *Poumon Coeur* 1983 Jan–Feb; 39(1): 53–7 (in French).]

27. The right supplements can keep your immune system strong

Biostim, a substance derived from a certain bacterium, can keep your immune system strong, especially when it's needed during bouts of infection like the flu. Studies have shown Biostim can protect those with compromised immune systems like the elderly and reduces the need to take large amounts of antibiotics. [Hugonot, R., Gutierrez, L.M., Hugonot, L. Preventive action of an immunomodulator on respiratory infections in elderly subjects. *Presse Med.* 1988 Jul 27; 17(28): 1445–9 (in French)]

28. Vitamins are essential for immune health

Low levels of nutrients like vitamins A, C, E and B6, copper, iron and zinc have been linked to immune dysfunction. Over the past three decades, science has repeatedly linked the connection between vitamin/mineral balance and proper immunity, infection resistance and allergy susceptibility. [High 1999, Johnson et all 1992, Grimble 1997, Shankar et al 1998, Ravaglia et al 2000]

29. Eat lots of carrots

Beta carotene boosts natural killer cell activity in elderly men. Researchers claim that eating vegetables high in beta carotene, like carrots, produces significantly greater production of certain immune system cells that fight infection. [Santos, M.S., Meydani, S.N., Leka, L., Wu, D., Fotouhi, N., Meydani, M., Hennekens,C.H., Gaziano, J.M. Natural killer cell activity in elderly men is enhanced by beta-carotene supplementation. *Am. J. Clin. Nutr.*1996; 64(5): 7727]

30. Beta carotene gives your immune system a boost

Studies show that longterm beta-carotene supplementation helps the immune system seek out viruses and bacteria. Because it is not known which types of carotenes are most beneficial, experts advise consuming many varieties. Beta-carotene enhances the killing capacity of natural killer cells in the immune system. [Carlos, T.F., Riondel, J., Mathieu, J., Guiraud, P., Mestries, J.C., Favier, A. Beta-carotene enhances natural killer cell activity in athymic mice. *In Vivo* 1997 Jan–Feb; 11(1): 87–91.]

31. Take more beta-carotene

Some studies have shown that this antioxidant does not necessarily increase the number of natural killer cells in our immune system. But it can significantly boost their killing capacity. NK cells attack and destroy unwanted pathogens in the body. [Carlos, T.F., Riondel, J., Mathieu, J., Guiraud, P., Mestries, J.C., Favier, A. Beta-carotene enhances natural killer cell activity in athymic mice. *In Vivo* 1997 Jan–Feb; 11(1): 87–91]

32. Increase your vitamin E intake

Long-term supplementation of vitamin E improves cell-mediated immunity. In fact, consuming doses larger than those recommended by the FDA showed stronger immune function in elderly people. This vitamin can help increase the power of the immune system, and help fight off invading organisms in the body. Supplementing with vitamin E for four months can improve cell-

mediated immunity. Taking doses larger than those currently rec-
ommended can enhance T-cell immune function in the elderly.
[Meydani, S.N., Meydani, M., Blumberg, J.B., Leka, L.S., Siber,
G., Loszewski, R.,Thompson, C., Pedrosa, M.C., Diamond, R.D.,
Stollar, B.D. Vitamin E supplementation and in vivo immune
response in healthy elderly subjects: a randomized controlled
trial. *JAMA* 1997; 277(17): 1380–6][Meydani, S.N., Meydani,
M., Blumberg, J.B., Leka, L.S., Siber, G., Loszewski, R.,Thompson,
C., Pedrosa, M.C., Diamond, R.D., Stollar, B.D. Vitamin E supple-
mentation and in vivo immune response in healthy elderly subjects:
a randomized controlled trial. [*JAMA* 1997; 277(17): 1380–6]

33. Don't forget your vitamin E
Consuming high dosages of vitamin E (alpha-tocopherol) supplements significantly increases killer cell activity, which attack invading organisms. There is a direct relationship between levels of
vitamin E and natural killer cell activity levels in the body. [Adachi,
N., Migita, M., Ohta, T., Higashi, A., Matsuda, I. Depressed natural killer cell activity due to decreased natural killer cell population
in a vitamin E-deficient patient with Shwachman syndrome:
reversible natural killer cell abnormality by alpha-tocopherol supplementation. *Eur. J. Pediatr.* 1997 Jun; 156(6): 444–8]

34. Vitamin E helps your heart
This essential vitamin not only boosts the immune system, but it
is crucial to cardiovascular health. Large amounts of vitamin E
may lower cholesterol levels and protect arteries from damage
caused by free radicals. But excessive amounts can have the
opposite effect [Pryor, W.A. Vitamin E and heart disease: basic
science to clinical intervention trials. *Free Radic. Biol. Med.* 2000
Jan 1; 28(1): 141–64]

35. Increase intake of vitamin E

Vitamin E, combined with the right mix of other vitamins and essential nutrients, can boost your immune system's ability to fight off infection. This nutrient, and others, are deficient in the American population. [Ravaglia, G., Forti, P., Maioli, F., Bastagli, L., Facchini, A., Mariani, E., Savarino, L., Sassi, S., Cucinotta, D., Lenaz, G. Effect of micronutrient status on natural killer cell immune function in healthy free-living subjects aged $>/= 90$ y. *Am. J. Clin. Nutr.* 2000 Feb; 71(2): 590–8]

36. Vitamin C is important

Consuming high levels of vitamin C may enhance vitamin E's ability to enhance the immune system. Vitamin C also helps clean up the free radicals that the immune system deposits following an oxidative burst killing activity. Because the body cannot manufacture nor store vitamin C, the best way to obtain this essential nutrient is to eat fruits, vegetables and take supplements. [Niki, E. Interaction of ascorbate and alpha-tocopherol. *Ann. N.Y. Acad. Sci.* 1987; 498: 186–99.]

37. Don't forget vitamin C

This vitamin can protect levels of vitamin E in tissue and may contribute to vitamin E's ability to boost the immune system. Vitamin C can also help wipe out free radicals after an immune system oxidative burst killing activity. [Stahl, W., Sies, H. Antioxidant defense: vitamins E and C and carotenoids. *Diabetes* 1997 Sep; 46(Suppl. 2): S14–8]

38. Increase intake of vitamin C

Vitamin C helps boost your healthy immune system. It interacts with other vitamins and minerals to help fight off disease.

88 Ways to Supercharge Your Immune System

[Shankar, A.H., Prasad, A.S. Zinc and immune function: the biological basis of altered resistance to infection. *Am. J. Clin. Nutr.* Aug 1998; 68(2 Suppl.): 447S–463S]

39. Vitamin B6 helps boost your immune system
Vitamin B6 (pyridoxine) helps boost immune system function. Deficiencies in this nutrient result in significantly lower levels of serum thymic factor, a hormone involved in cell-mediated immunity. [Chandra, S., Chandra, R.K. Nutrition, immune response, and outcome. *Prog. Food Nutr. Sci.* 1986; 10(1–2): 1–65]

40. Don't forget vitamin B6
Animal studies have shown that low levels of vitamin B6 in the body lead to suppression of the immune system. The vitamin directly activates enzymes needed to maintain your immune system's healthy function during attacks against unwanted invaders. [Rall, L.C., Meydani, S.N. Vitamin B6 and immune competence. *Nutr. Rev.* 1993 Aug; 51(8): 217–25.] Infants, young children and pregnant or nursing women face a high risk of zinc deficiency. Populations like atopic, formula-fed children, low-birth-weight infants, obese adolescents, malnourished hospital patients, and the elderly generally have comprised immune systems, and face increased risk of infection and allergic disorders. These conditions and diseases can be corrected with the proper consumption of certain nutrients and foods. [Chandra, R.K. Nutrition and immunology: from the clinic to cellular biology and back again. *Proc. Nutr. Soc.* 1999 Aug; 58(3): 681–3.]

41. Remember to take vitamin B6
Not only can this vitamin enhance immunity, it has many healthy functions in the body. Deficits of vitamin B6 can lead to a signif-

icant lowering of serum thymic factor, a hormone involved in the immune function. [Katunuma, N., Matsui, A., Endo, K., Hanba, J., Sato, A., Nakano, M., Yuto, Y., Tada, Y., Asao, T., Himeno, K., Maekawa, Y., Inubushi, T. Inhibition of intracellular cathepsin activities and suppression of immune responses mediated by helper T lymphocyte type-2 by peroral or intraperitoneal administration of vitamin B6. *Biochem. Biophys. Res. Commun.* 2000 May 27; 272(1): 151–5]

42. Zinc fights toxic heavy metals in your body
Trace elements are necessary in our diet, not only for their antioxidant activity, but also for efficient wound healing and immune function. These trace elements are greatly affected by so-called heavy metals like aluminum, arsenic, cadmium, lead and mercury. Zinc consumption helps ward off the negative effect of cadmium on natural killer cell activity in the body. [Chowdhury, B.A., Chandra, R.K. Biological and Health Implications of Toxic Heavy Metal and Essential Trace Element Interactions. *Prog. Food Nutr. Sci.* 1987; 11(1): 55–113.]

43. Zinc helps keep your cells healthy
The trace element zinc has many roles in the efficient function of cells, including cell division and activation. Zinc also functions as an antioxidant and stabilizes cell membranes. [Prasad, A.S. Effects of zinc deficiency on Th1 and Th2 cytokine shifts. *J. Infect Dis.* 2000 Sep; 182(Suppl. 1): S62–S68.]

44. Zinc helps you maintain your resistance
Deficiencies in the trace element zinc result in reduced resistance to infection. When disease-causing organisms invade, studies have shown that low levels of zinc help the invading parasite survive better. [Scott, M.E., Koski, K.G. Zinc deficiency impairs

immune responses against parasitic nematode infections at intestinal and systemic sites. *J. Nutr.* 2000 May; 130(5S Suppl.): 1412S–20S.]

45. Remember to take your zinc

Levels of zinc affect levels of beneficial immune system proteins known as cytokines, but have no effect on anti-inflammatory cytokines. Zinc deficiency also results in decreased production of beneficial cytokines and interleukins, as well as lower levels of T-cells, which oversee the attack of invading organisms. [Prasad, A.S. Effects of zinc deficiency on Th1 and Th2 cytokine shifts. *J. Infect Dis.* 2000 Sep; 182 (Suppl. 1): S62–S68]

46. Zinc and selenium fight infection

Seniors who take modest doses of a supplement containing zinc and selenium can significantly reduce the threat of infection, as well as the need for antibiotics. The mix of these two essential nutrients can help keep your immune system healthy and strong. [Chandra, R.K. Effect of vitamin and trace-element supplementation on immune responses and infection in elderly subjects. *Lancet* 1992 Nov 7; 340(8828): 1124–7; comment, *Lancet* 1993 Jan 30; 341(8840): 306–7]

47. Increase your intake of Zinc

Studies have shown that elderly people who take combinations of zinc and selenium give their immune system a boost. Seniors who take modest doses of supplements that contain these trace elements generally lower their susceptibility to infection, as well as their need for antibiotics. [Chandra, R.K. Effect of Vitamin and Trace-Element Supplementation on Immune Responses and Infection in Elderly Subjects. *Lancet* 1992 Nov 7; 340(8828): 1124–7; comment, *Lancet* 1993 Jan 30; 341(8840): 306–7.]

48. Keep your infection risk low by taking Zinc

Seniors who consume combinations of zinc and selenium wind up with significantly lower risk of infection. This combination of trace elements improves antibody response to flu vaccine. [Girodon, F. Galan, P. Monget, A.L., Boutron-Ruault, M.C., Brunet-Lecomte, P., Preziosi, P., Arnaud, J., Manuguerra, J.C., Herchberg, S. Impact of Trace Elements and Vitamin Supplementation on Immunity and Infections in Institutionalized Elderly Patients: A Randomized Controlled Trial. MIN. VIT. AOX. geriatric network. *Arch. Intern. Med.* 1999 Apr 12; 159(7): 748–54.]

49. Keeping a healthy GI system

Conditions like lactose intolerance, food allergy, gluten insensitivity, ulcerative colitis, and Crohn's disease will cause the gut lining to become "leaky". This allows incompletely digested food proteins to enter the bloodstream, prompting an immune system inflammatory response. If the condition is not corrected at the source, this immune response can become chronic, leading to further damage. Only a diet rich in certain nutrients can protect against this risk, but it is necessary to combine a balanced group of nutrients to achieve these benefits. [Lesourd, B.M. Nutrition and immunity in the elderly: modification of immune responses with nutritional treatments. *Am. J. Clin. Nutr.* 1997 Aug; 66(2): 478S–484S.] Probiotics are substances that can enhance the bacteria flora of the intestinal tract. One such probiotic, lactobacillus acidophilus, is found in live yogurt cultures and can fight yeast and other unwanted organisms found in the GI tract. Another probiotic, bifidobacterium lactis, is found in low-lactose milk and can improve immune function. [Arunachalam, K., Gill, H.S., Chandra, R.K. Enhancement of natural immune function by dietary consumption of *Bifidobacterium lactis* (HN019). *Eur. J. Clin. Nutr.* 2000 Mar; 54(3): 263–7.]

50. Maintain a healthy GI system
In the gut, a thinning of cells that make up its essential lining can cause toxins to leak into the bloodstream. This can happen when changes in cellular structure result. [Hunter, J.O. Food allergy— or enterometabolic disorder. [*Lancet* 1991 Aug 24; 338(8765): 495–6]

51. Boost your GI system's immune capability
Probiotics like lactobacillus acidophilus, lactobacillus bulgaricus and lactobacillus casei can enhance the immune response in the GI tract. They can also maintain gut flora balance and enhance nutrient formation for intestinal cells called enterocytes. [Chiang, B.L., Sheih, Y.H., Wang, L.H., Liao, C.K., Gill, H.S. Enhancing Immunity by Dietary Consumption of a Probiotic Lactic Acid Bacterium (*Bifidobacterium lactis* HN019): Optimization and Definition of Cellular Immune Responses. *Eur. J. Clin. Nutr.* 2000 Nov; 54(11): 849–55.]

52. Maintain a strong and healthy GI system
Lactoferin is a prebiotic substance that promotes the production of beneficial probiotics that enhance immunity in the GI tract. Lactoferin also discourages formation of antagonistic bacteria and is naturally found in many mucous membrane secretions in the body, suggesting a natural immune enhancing ability. [Nishiya, K., Horwitz, D.A. Contrasting effects of lactoferrin on human lymphocyte and monocyte natural killer activity and anti-body-dependent cell-mediated cytotoxicity. *J. Immunol.* 1982 Dec; 129(6): 2519–23.]

53. Keep unwanted bacteria away from your GI tract

Lactoferrin is beneficial for the immune system. It indirectly increases immune response in the GI tract and discourages the growth of harmful bacteria like E-coli, Staphylococci, and H. pylori. [Wada, T., Aiba, Y., Shimizu, K., Takagi, A., Miwa, T., Koga, Y. The therapeutic effect of bovine lactoferrin in the host infected with *Helicobacter pylori*. *Scand. J. Gastroenterol.* 1999 Mar; 34(3): 238–43.]

54. Watch the type of fats you consume

The types of fat people consume determine the balance of pro-inflammatory and anti-inflammatory hormones and messengers linked to the immune response. Polyunsaturated fatty acids are absorbed into cell membranes and influence the cell's various biological responses. Fatlike substances known as lipids help keep your cells stable and healthy. Consumption of linoleic acid can dramatically promote the growth of tumors, whereas fatty acids like linolenic and eicosapentaenoic acids can fight cancer. [Penturf, M.E., McGlone, J.J., Griswold, J.A. Lipopolysaccharide-induced enhancement of natural killer cell cytotoxicity: comparison of rats fed menhaden, safflower and essential fatty acid deficient diets. *J. Nutr. Immunol.* 1997; 5(2): 47–56.]

55. Certain kinds of fats are good for you

Omega-3 fatty acids reduces the risk of cardiovascular diseases like arrhythmia and hypertension, protects against renal disease, improves symptoms of rheumatoid arthritis, and protects against infection. Different fatty acids, in general, have different effects on various cells of the immune system. [Sauer, L.A., Dauchy, R.T., Blask, D.E. *Mechanism for the Antitumor and Anticachetic Effects of n-3 Fatty Acids* 2001. Cooperstown, NY: Bassett

Research Institute (lensauer@juno.com).]

56. Omega-3 fatty acids are essential

Omega-3 fatty acids help keep your immune system in check. Consumption of omega-3 fatty acids can reduce the risk of cardiovascular diseases, renal disease, rheumatoid arthritis progression, inflammatory bowel diseases, and can protect against infection. [Sauer, L.A., Dauchy, R.T., Blask, D.E. *Mechanism for the Antitumor and Anticachetic Effects of n-3 Fatty Acids* 2001. Cooperstown, NY: Bassett Research Institute (lensauer@juno.com).]

57. Remember to take Echinacea

Echinacea, a member of the daisy family, is commonly used to prevent and treat the common cold and other upper respiratory infections. It is also effective against urinary tract and vaginal yeast infections. [See, D.M., Broumand, N., Sahl, L., Tilles, J.G. In vitro effects of echinacea and ginseng on natural killer and antibody-dependent cell cytotoxicity in healthy subjects and chronic fatigue syndrome or acquired immunodeficiency syndrome patients. *Immunopharmacology* Jan 1997; 35(3): 229–35.]

58. Don't forget to take Echinacea

Echinacea fights respiratory infections, increases antibody production, reduces inflammation and augments white blood cells' ability to travel to sites of infection. This extract can also fight urinary tract and yeast infections. [See, D.M., Broumand, N., Sahl, L., Tilles, J.G. In vitro effects of echinacea and ginseng on natural killer and antibody-dependent cell cytotoxicity in healthy subjects and chronic fatigue syndrome or acquired immunodeficiency syndrome patients. *Immunopharmacology* Jan 1997; 35(3): 229–35]

59. Echinacea boosts your immune system

A derivative of echinacea, echinacea purpurea, contains chemicals found in many plants that stimulate production of natural killer cells that make up the immune system. This supplement also helps prevent natural killer cell breakdown function in older animals. [Currier, N.L., Miller, S.C. Natural killer cells from aging mice treated with extracts from *Echinacea purpurea* are quantitatively and functionally rejuvenated. *Exp. Gerontol.* 2000 Aug; 35(5): 627–39.]

60. Echinacea and ginseng have combined benefits

Both Echinacea purpurea and Panax ginseng stimulates the production of immune system cells, especially in those with chronic fatigue syndrome or AIDS. These extracts showed significant effects as well, in people with depressed cellular immunity. [See D.M., Broumand, N., Sahl, L., Tilles, J.G. In vitro effects of echinacea and ginseng on natural killer and antibody-dependent cell cytotoxicity in healthy subjects and chronic fatigue syndrome or acquired immunodeficiency syndrome patients. *Immunopharmacology* Jan 1997; 35(3): 229–35]

61. Remember to take your Ginseng

Ginseng has been used as a powerful medicine for some 2,000 years. This supplement—combined with multivitamins and minerals—is more effective than multivitamins and minerals alone in improving quality of life for people who face lots of stress. [Caso, M.A, Vargas Ruiz, R., Salas Villagomez, A., Begona Infante, C. Double-blind study of a multivitamin complex supplemented with ginseng extract. *Drugs Exp. Clin. Res.* 1996; 22(6): 323–9.]

62. Why Ginseng is so important

Panax ginseng significantly reduces the risk of the common cold and influenza. This supplement is effective when started one month prior to influenza vaccination and continued for eight subsequent weeks. [Scaglione, F., Cattaneo, G., Alessandria, M., Cogo, R. Efficacy and safety of the standardised Ginseng extract G115 for potentiating vaccination against the influenza syndrome and protection against the common cold [corrected]. *Drugs Exp. Clin. Res.* 1996; 22(2): 65–72.]

63. Ginseng can help ease stress

Ginseng taken in combination with multivitamins and minerals is more effective than vitamins and minerals alone in improving the quality of life in high-stress people. American ginseng is used as an adaptogen, a compound that helps the body adapt to stress. [Scaglione, F., Cattaneo, G., Alessandria, M., Cogo, R. Efficacy and safety of the standardised Ginseng extract G115 for potentiating vaccination against the influenza syndrome and protection against the common cold [corrected]. *Drugs Exp. Clin. Res.* 1996; 22(2): 65–72]

64. Increase your antioxidant consumption

The supplement known as grape seed-skin extract provides antioxidant benefits 50 times greater than vitamin E and 20 times greater than vitamin C. A substance found in grape seed-skin extract, proanthocyanidins, has been shown in research to boost production of beneficial immune system proteins like interleukin-2 [Bagchi, D., Garg, A., Krohn, R.L., Bagchi, M., Tran, M.X., Stohs, S.J. Oxygen free radical scavenging abilities of vitamins C and E, and a grape seed proanthocyanidin extract in vitro. *Res. Commun. Mol. Pathol. Pharmacol.* 1997 Feb; 95(2): 179–89.]

65. Consuming the right ingredients may help fight cancer

The compound known as MGN-3 significantly increases the immune system's ability to fight cancer. It could be used as a new biological response modifier with possible implications for cancer. [Ghoneum, M. Enhancement of human natural killer cell activity by modified arabinoxylane from rice bran (MGN-3). *Int. J. Immunother.* 1998; 14(2): 89–99.]

66. Take whey protein to detoxify harmful substances

Whey protein isolate dramatically raises levels of glutathione, a substance that protects immune cells and detoxifies harmful compounds in the body. Reduced glutathione levels have been linked to AIDS and other viral diseases. Raising levels of this substance appears to be one method of modulating immunity. [Micke, P., Beeh, K.M., Schlaak, J.F., Buhl, R. Oral supplementation with whey proteins increases plasma glutathione levels of HIV-infected patients. *Eur. J. Clin. Invest.* 2001 Feb; 31(2): 171–8.]

67. Take whey protein to help ward off tumors

Doses of whey protein concentrate decrease tumor prevalence and reduce pooled areas of tumors known as tumor mass index. This protein provides a greater beneficial effect than other proteins, including soy. [McIntosh, G.H., Regester, G.O., Le Leu, R.K., Royle, P.J., Smithers, G.W. Dairy proteins protect against dimethylhydrazine-induced intestinal cancers in rats. *J. Nutr.* 1995 Apr; 125(4): 809–16.]

68. Take carnitine to help your immune system fight off invaders

High doses of carnitine appear to increase natural killer cell activity in the immune system. This amino acid, found mainly in meats, transports fat across the cellular membrane and breaks down fat within cells. It has implications in combating AIDS. [Franceschi, C., Cossarizza, A., Troiano, L., Salati, R., Monti, D. Immunological parameters in aging: studies on natural immuno-modulatory and immunoprotective substances. *Int. J. Clin. Pharmacol. Res.* 1990; 10(1–2): 53–7.]

69. Take CoQ10 to keep your heart strong and arteries healthy

Coenzyme Q10 improves quality of life for people with advanced heart disease, congestive heart failure, angina and arrhythmia. It increases a number of immune system cells including IgG and T4 cells. [Folkers, K., Morita, M., McRee, J., Jr. The activities of coenzyme Q10 and vitamin B6 for immune responses. *Biochem. Biophys. Res. Commun.* 1993 May 28; 193(1): 88–92.]

70. CoQ10 is important as a cancer preventive

Coenzyme Q10 is a powerful adjuvant therapy for people with various types of cancer. It has been shown to significantly reduce metastases and lower the risk of death in breast cancer patients. [Lockwood, K., Moesgaard, S., Folkers, K. Partial and complete regression of breast cancer in patients in relation to dosage of coenzyme Q10. *Biochem. Biophys. Res. Commun.* 1994a Mar 30; 199(3): 1504–8.]

71. Take supplements containing DHEA to fight the effects of aging

DHEA is a steroid hormone produced in the adrenal gland. Supplemental DHEA has been shown to provide anti-aging, anti-obesity and anti-cancer influences, as well as a significant ability to enhance the immune system through several different mechanisms. [Danenberg, H.D., Ben-Yehuda, A., Zakay-Rones, Z., Friedman, G. Dehydroepiandrosterone (DHEA) treatment reverses the impaired immune response of old mice to influenza vaccination and protects from influenza infection. *Vaccine* 1995; 13(15): 1445–8.]

72. DHEA is extremely beneficial for older adults

In older adults, DHEA supplementation fights aging, boosts the number of immune cells, increases the number of B immune cell and B-cell activity, increases production of beneficial immune system proteins like interleukin-2, and boosts the number of natural killer cells, as well as other components of the immune system. [Khorram, O., Vu, L., Yen, S.S. Activation of immune function by dehydro-epiandrosterone (DHEA) in age-advanced men. *J. Gerontol. A Biol. Sci. Med. Sci.* 1997 Jan; 52(1): M1–7.]

73. Take DHEA to help fight off disease

DHEA boosts beneficial immune system proteins like interleukin-2 and decreases levels of damaging interleukin-6, which is believed to play a key role in diseases like rheumatoid arthritis, osteoporosis, arteriosclerosis and late-onset B-cell neoplasia. DHEA also suppresses several detrimental immune components, reducing the risk of heart failure, osteoporosis, arthritis, and dementia. [Ferrucci, L., Harris, T.B., Guralnik, J.M., Tracy, R.P.,

Corti, M.C., Cohen, H.J., Penninx, B., Pahor, M., Wallace, R., Havlik, R.J. Serum IL-6 level and the development of disability in older persons. *J. Am. Geriatr. Soc.* 1999 Jun; 47(6): 639–46; comment, *J. Am. Geriatr. Soc.* 1999 Jun; 47(6): 755–6.]

74. Take DHEA to keep your immune system strong

DHEA boosts production of a key immune system protein known as interleukin-2 and other beneficial immune components. At the same time, it suppresses interleukin-6 and other detrimental immune components, and has been shown to be effective against a disease known as lupus erythematosus. [van Vollenhoven, R.F., Morabito, L.M., Engleman, E.G., McGuire, J.L. Treatment of systemic lupus erythematosus with dehydroepiandrosterone: 50 patients treated up to 12 months. *J. Rheumatol.* 1998 Feb; 25(2): 28–59.]

75. Keep nutritional supplements that contain DHEA handy

DHEA keeps cytokine production at normal levels, which helps stave off the effects of aging. The hormone also increases levels of beneficial immune system proteins. [Inserra, P., Zhang, Z., Ardestani, S.K., Araghi-Niknam, M. Liang, B., Jiang, S., Shaw, D., Molitor, M., Elliott, K., Watson, R.R. Modulation of cytokine production by dehydroepiandrosterone (DHEA) plus melatonin (MLT) supplementation of old mice. *Proc. Soc. Exp. Biol. Med.* 1998 May; 218(1): 76–82.]

76. DHEA is a key supplement for good health

DHEA restores normal production of cytokines, proteins inherent for the normal function of cells. At the same time, it inhibits production of "bad" proteins that are bad for your health. [Inserra, P., Zhang, Z., Ardestani, S.K., Araghi-Niknam, M.

Liang, B., Jiang, S., Shaw, D., Molitor, M., Elliott, K., Watson, R.R. Modulation of cytokine production by dehydroepiandrosterone (DHEA) plus melatonin (MLT) supplementation of old mice. *Proc. Soc. Exp. Biol. Med.* 1998 May; 218(1): 76–82.]

77. Keep nutritional supplements on hand
Melatonin improves immune function by increasing production of cells that attack microbial invaders. Melatonin also enhances production of natural killer cells and essential immune system proteins. [Lissoni, P., Barni, S., Crispino, S., Tancini, G., Fraschini, F. Endocrine and immune effects of melatonin therapy in metastatic cancer patients. *Eur. J. Cancer Clin. Oncol.* 1989 May; 25(5): 789–95].

78. Working out helps fight disease
Studies show regular physical activity may boost production of natural killer cells which make up part of your immune system. These NK cells attack and destroy invading organisms in the body. [Shinkai, S., Konishi, M., Shephard, R.J. Aging, exercise, training, and the immune system. *Exerc. Immunol. Rev.* 1997; 3: 68–95]

79. Balance a good diet with an effective workout program
Scientists have discovered that diets very low in fat combined with a strenuous exercise regimen can decrease immune system effectiveness. Take vitamins to replace any nutrients you may not gain from your diet. [Venkatraman, J.T., Rowland, J.A., Denardin, E., Horvath, P.J., Pendergast, D.R. Influence of level of dietary lipids and exercise on immune status in athletes. *FASEB J.* 1996; 10(3): A556]

80. Don't forget vitamin A

Vitamin A boosts cellular communication and maintains the integrity of the body's mucosal surfaces. It also protects against tumor growth, and helps maintain a feeling of overall good health. [Villamor, E., Fawzi, W.W. Vitamin A supplementation: implications for morbidity and mortality in children. *J. Infect. Dis.* 2000 Sep; 182(Suppl.1): S122–S133]

81. Increase your intake of vitamin A

Vitamin A is the anti-infective vitamin. It has been shown that vitamin A protects against tumor growth. In addition to its abilities as a cell-signaling vitamin, it maintains the integrity of the body's mucosal surfaces. [Villamor E, Fawzi W.W. Vitamin A supplementation: implications for morbidity and mortality in children. *J Infect Dis* 2000 Sep; 182(Suppl. 1): S122–S123]

82. Remember to eat your spinach

Spinach contains beta-carotene, an antioxidant that has a powerful effect in boosting the immune system's natural killer cells. Studies have shown beta-carotene has a dramatic effect on the immune system in elderly men. [Santos, M.S., Meydani, S.N., Leka, L., Wu, D., Fotouhi, N., Meydani, M., Hennekens, C.H., Gaziano, J.M. Natural killer cell activity in elderly men is enhanced by beta-carotene supplementation. *Am. J. Clin. Nutr.* 1996; 64(5): 772–7]

83. Trace elements are essential

Trace elements contain powerful antioxidant properties. They enhance wound healing and immune activity. Dietary supplements of trace elements replace the depleted minerals in the food we eat. [Chowdhury, B.A., Chandra, R.K. Biological and health implications of toxic heavy metal and essential trace element interactions. *Prog. Food Nutr. Sci.* 1987; 11(1): 55–113]

84. Increase your intake of lactoferrin

This substance suppresses the buildup of unwanted bacteria. Lactoferrin is found in many mucous membrane secretions, suggesting that it may have the ability to boost immune system function. [Nishiya, K., Horwitz, D.A. Contrasting effects of lactoferrin on human lymphocyte and monocyte natural killer activity and antibody-dependent cell-mediated cytotoxicity. *J. Immunol.* 1982 Dec; 129(6): 2519–23]

85. MGN-3 boosts your body's infection-fighting ability

MGN-3, a substance produced by hydrolyzing rice bran, improves natural killer cell activity, inhibits tumor growth. Some studies suggest MGN-3 may enhance NK cell production in cancer. [Ghoneum, M., Namatalla, G. NK Immunomodulatory Function in 27 Cancer Patients by MGN-3, a Modified Arabinoxylane from Rice Bran. 87th Annual Meeting of the American Association for Cancer Research, April 20–24, 1996 (Abstr.).]

86. Keep your cortisol levels in check

High doses of the European procaine drug KH3 can protect against elevated cortisol levels in the body. Cortisol is a damaging hormone that is seen in cancer, AIDS, and high stress levels. KH3 also indirectly boosts the immune system by lowering cortisol levels. Melatonin combined with DHEA can help suppress cortisol levels, as well. They also enhance production of several immune system cells and beneficial proteins. [Maestroni, G.J. The immunoneuroendocrine role of melatonin. *J. Pineal Res.* 1993 Jan; 14(1): 1–10]

87. Help fight infections with Biostim

Biostim is an immunomodulator extracted from a bacterium. It can reduce the number and duration of a range of infections. Biostim can also prevent infections, as well as the need for antibiotics, during cold and flu season. [Viallat, J.R., Costantini, D., Boutin, C., Farisse, P. Double-blind study of an immunomodulator of bacterial origin (Biostim) in the prevention of infectious episodes in chronic bronchitis. *Poumon Coeur* 1983 Jan–Feb; 39(1): 53–7 (in French).]

88. Combine exercise with proper nutrients

Vitamin supplementation combined with exercise is essential because physical activity boosts oxygen demand, causing an increase in the formation of oxygen radical species. Many vitamins, however, act as an energy metabolizer and free radical scavenger. While you exercise, watch what you eat. A very low fat diet combined with a strenuous workout schedule can be detrimental to the immune system. [Konig, D., Berg, A., Weinstock, C., Keul, J., Northoff, H. Essential fatty acids, immune function, and exercise. *Exerc. Immunol. Rev.* 1997; 3: 1–31]

8

POSITIVE AFFIRMATIONS

ONE of the most important steps we can take in caring of ourselves is to keep our mind focused on what is possible. We can and must focus on becoming whole. Otherwise, we will forever be honoring the world of disinformation, distortion, and lies that work against us.

The vast majority of Americans are conscientious, hardworking and do their darndest to try to play by the rules. The trouble is that the rules are manipulated so that the person rarely has a chance to survive and thrive with happiness and fulfillment. More often than not, the rules are made by people who lead us to spend money we don't have, to buy things we don't need and to create debt we can't afford. To manage the resulting stress, they provide us with sublimating activities that cause further victimization—gambling, drugs, alcohol, pornography, compulsive working and medication. So other people create our problems and people then manipulate our solutions.

If we're ready to change and fill that emptiness within our lives with meaning, then we have to know that our lives count, that we do not have to accept everyone else's advice or live by their reality. There is a purpose to our existence. We honor that purpose by accepting, affirming, and focusing on it by having positive goals. By so doing, we can regain what is essentially ours.

With this in mind, I have created some affirmations. All I ask is that each day your read a single affirmation and continue to look at it throughout the day. Whenever there is a problem, remind yourself that life is dualistic. For every negative there is a positive, for every crisis a blissful moment, for every breakdown a breakthrough. These affirmations are meant to offer balance in a world that appears to be toxic and out of balance.

1. People who ultimately succeed in life generally have made many more mistakes than other people, but they don't view the mistake as a traumatic endpoint. Mistakes are seen, instead, as launching pads for learning. Edison, the inventor, is a classic example of this technique in which mistakes are welcomed as teachers. The light bulb, now the universal symbol for a brilliant new idea, was perfected only after thousands of errors led Edison patiently to its discovery. Never give up!

2. I have never seen a situation that was so bad that being positive couldn't improve something in that situation. Positive energy yields solutions; negative energy never does.

This is a true story. During World War II, a group of Jewish women arrived at Auschwitz. They were told to form one line. At the front of this line stood one of Hitler's SS commanders with a baton. If the baton pointed to the right, the woman could work and her life was spared. If the baton pointed to the left, the woman was infirm or too old to work, and she would be killed.

A plain young woman with a withered hand came next in line before the captain. In a small but brave voice, she said, " Good morning, sir." A moment passed as he looked at the woman's useless hand. Another moment. "Yes, it is a good morning," he replied. In a flash, the baton firmly pointed to the right! She was spared because of one life-affirming "Good morning!" Yes, positive energy does yield positive solutions!

3. That which creates comfort can create complacency. Complacency stops the growth process. The mother bear hibernates comfortably all winter in the grip of passivity, but she does not grow. To grow she must awaken and abandon the security of her cave to find food. She must return to the world and the needs of her cubs. So must you. Your world family needs you.

4. When you live in each moment, life is simple. We complicate life with our preconceived notions, and then we wonder why we are so often disappointed.

5. Do you volunteer to be a victim? Does this bring you redemption, love, just sympathy, or ultimately rejection when people get tired of hearing about your troubles? Can you see the cycle of self-hatred here? Has your desperate need for attention led you to seek out insults to complain about? Stop blaming. Start growing.

6. Has your stuff become more important than your life? Do you lose sleep worrying about your car? Has your computer, a robot, replaced your best friend? Have you had your cell phone surgically attached to your ear so you won't miss a call from your computer? If so, it's time to pare down to the bare essentials of life. Go camping! Leave that T.V. home! Lighten your load. Downsize to make life simple again.

7. Don't allow someone else to control how you feel. No one should have the power to make you miserable unless you secretly welcome the misery. We like to star in our own dramas.

8. Your best education comes through life—especially

through making mistakes, being humiliated, feeling stupid, and being embarrassed. Now don't run after these They find all of us for our own benefit, so we won't take ourselves too seriously and go around hurting people with our arrogance and inflated egos.

9. Much of what we think, feel and do every day is based on pre-conditioned notions. When you cling to fixed expectations (automatic pilot), you are bound to be disappointed and to become upset frequently. For example, if you believe that everyone you know must greet you with a smile, you're setting yourself up for what you perceive as insults, followed by fear, grief and anger. This is self-sabotage. Live more in the moment.

10. I thought that if I could do enough, I'd be enough. I did more than enough, but I don't feel like I am enough. I am sacred. I do not have to do anything; by just being alive, I am enough.

11. Do you fear change? Why? What happens when you are forced to change? What happens when you choose something? You have to be responsible for the choice you make. Actually, greed also partly explains our fear to commit to a choice. Think of all the options we lose when we favor just one.

12. Be responsible for your actions. Criminals take all the credit when they get away with something, but they never want to take the blame when they get caught. "Incorrigibles" are often raised in homes or on streets where mischief is rewarded subtly at an early age. The message is, "Get away with as much as you can." Disgrace is getting nailed for a crime. The crime itself is winked at in this mindset. Are you winking at crime?—Flirting with inflicting suffering on oth-

ers is a dangerous game. Taking responsibility for your actions is more a step toward growth.

13. You don't tackle a crisis by just addressing the symptoms. You deal with the causes.

14. Do your actions and lifestyle reflect your inner beliefs?

15. How can you get involved and help people without becoming a victim in the process?—It's about sacrifice! I must accept that there are sacrifices that will occur in all service, but they needn't be fatal.

16. Are you a person who waits for things to change, or do you make things change? How little comes to you if you are waiting! Everything is there; find it. There is little probability that things are going to interfere in your life to make it better. You are fully responsible for that. So stop waiting for things to change. Change them!

17. You're not going to change society by changing yourself to be accepted by society. Your unique contribution, which may be to rebel and correct, will be lost forever if you take the more comfortable road and adapt. You will have lost your mission!

18. Make your most important decisions in a positive frame of mind.

A positive frame of mind must be cultivated, much as you would prepare a field to receive seeds. It is unrealistic to expect a positive or receptive mindset to overtake you just because you need it at decision time. Rather, consider the style of President Abraham Lincoln who had prepared himself to make certain life and death decisions by determining in advance that the protection of the greatest number of people is required for a wise decision. This was his foundation.

Many deserters were court-martialed during our Civil War and

President Lincoln was often beseeched by relatives of deserters to pardon them. He would accept almost any reason to do so. His positive frame of mind told him that there were enough weeping widows and orphans without his creating more by killing men who had made errors in judgment by running from responsibility. One general in particular who had many deserters in his ranks begged Lincoln to let deserters die on the premise that setting deserters free would be unfair to the soldiers who stayed and fought. Lincoln refused him vehemently because his positive frame of mind was set to keep bloodshed to a minimum.

However, it must be noted that when a slave-trader was sentenced to death, Lincoln staunchly refused to commute his sentence, stating that the man had stolen Africa's people from their homeland and forced them and their children to work here for generations in misery as slaves. A decision to pardon this man was unthinkable to Lincoln because his positive mindset told him that this slave-trader had gone out of his way to harm whole families of innocent people for material gain. This was odious to Lincoln because it was in direct opposition to Lincoln's own positive philosophy of protecting both the majority and minority when possible. Lincoln's decisions were always consistent with his positive foundation. Do you have a positive foundation for your decisions?

19. Life is a series of passages, through which all people assist us.
20. We remember the best experience of our lives and we look around to see if it will happen again, and it rarely does. Can you look at each experience with fresh eyes?
21. What we deny, we cannot change.
22. We should only have to hear something that is important once.

23. The more prepared you are, the more open you are, the more opportunities will come to you.
24. When you have used love to meet a challenge and to overcome an obstacle, you are connected to your bliss.
25. The present allows you to have a non-conflict moment. When you are present, you'll make no excuses for the past. You will no longer use the negative experiences from yesterday to deny you the completeness of today,
26. If you need someone to love you, it means you need someone else to validate you. You are depending on another for your self-esteem.
27. People confuse what they do with who they are. You are more relevant than your work or possessions.
28. None of us has complete control over what happens to us. Live as if today counts.
29. We must be open to ideas that challenge our own beliefs in order to grow.
30. If your relationship does not honor your needs, then reevaluate why you're still trying to make it work. What are you trying to prove?
31. Not to do something is also a conscious choice.
32. Wisdom transcends knowledge.
33. When we receive praise or respect from others, we tell ourselves that others like us. This is what happens when we are externally driven by what we do to create our reality. We have to ask ourselves if we would like ourselves without the recognition of others.
34. We tend to base too much in our lives on external realities.
35. We should ask ourselves what we have sacrificed spiritually in order to have our standard of living.
36. We cling to permanent religious beliefs, permanent social

beliefs and permanent political beliefs.

37. Think of the things in our lives we want to keep forever. We want our kids to be kids forever, and then one day everyone grows up. Much of our anxiety comes from the anger we feel because we've lost the present moment by focusing our energy on the past or on the future. We're so preoccupied with gaining something from the future that we lose what we have in the present. By looking forward, how can you know where you are? Live in this moment.

38. All we have is this moment, nothing else.

39. Most people want more than the moment. We want to recapture the moment, which we cannot do. To paraphrase a Greek philosopher, "You can never step twice into the same river." That is because no two seconds in a river's history are the same. It may take the same course, but every drop of water flowing by is different. What we have to appreciate is that every moment of every day of our lives is different. No two kisses are the same. No two meals are the same. Your joy comes from just being in this unique moment.

40. How can I honor my inner self if my whole world is based on my external self? The truth is there is no self.

41. Everything you do is a choice; not to do is its opposite.

42. The ego binds the intellect.

43. It is only the internal process that allows us to understand the external in which we live.

44. A "joy journal" lets us know that something we thought or did or shared with someone was so important to us that we found utter joy in it. It's important to see how much joy we are allowing into our lives.

45. Look for a person who is healthy and happy, and then ask

them for some guidance.

46. There is a difference between your conditioned wants and your essential needs. Only allow into your life what is really missing.
47. The only thing that is uniquely yours is your time.
48. Listen to someone without being the critic. Listen neutrally and learn.
49. We like to believe that people are all the same. No one is the same as anyone else. Everyone is different. We don't honor our differences. We like to collectivize people.

   It is a fascinating fact that no two human bodies are identical. Each human heart is shaped just a bit differently, the pattern of the arteries varies; the contours of the livers are not the same; the kidneys are never suspended in quite the same way.

   Immunity also varies from person to person. Two people may walk down the same street and get stung on their left thumbs by two bees. The first person barely gets a welt out of it and in two hours, the second person is dead.

   The fact that each human body is unique means that each of us occupies a special position on this earth. No one can replace another.

Let us refuse to allow the persistent procession of individuals who appear before us throughout our lives to melt into one anonymous mass of faceless flesh! With all our strength, we must reject the notion that people and groups of people are all alike and that they can be racially and ethnically pigeon-holed, disrespected, and computerized into mathematical symbols, giving them the status of nothing but a number!

50. Time is the same for everyone. It's what we do with it that makes a difference.

51. Accept everyone as being beautiful until they show that he or she is not.

52. Trust that everything you need to express and everything you need to communicate is already in place. All you have to do is get out of the way and allow it to express itself.

53. Honor and enjoy what you have! Appreciation is the secret of true success—the kind you cannot lose.

54. In our world, we have learned to gain at someone else's loss. Is that inhumane?

55. How many times in your life have you set a goal that no one could achieve? Be realistic. Set goals slightly above your comfort zone to create discomfort in order to grow. Remember the oyster and pearl!

56. We like to think we are something that we are not to compensate for our fear of being inadequate as we are.

57. No matter where you run, you take your negative thoughts with you. Try traveling light instead. Surrender your mind to the moment. Let the moment win your full attention! The sun is rising to distract you from your negative thoughts! The whole universe is charged with this compassionate mission to rescue you from your busy mind!

58. You've made success more important than happiness. Happiness is a real emotion, but success can be an illusion.

59. Sometimes we work so hard to be someplace else; we don't pay attention to the present. This is how we lose the appreciation of the beauty in our lives!

60. Surrender your ego! Violence and the need for rigid control will die with it!

61. When you realize that other people do have a right to a life, then they become sacred to you. We all like to be loved,

honored and recognized.

62. Dynamic people live by challenges. It's only through challenge that you're forced to use your strengths. Challenge brings out the best in us. So why don't you bring challenge into your everyday life? Live by challenge!

63. Your thoughts create fear. How you've been conditioned determines how you are going to bring your thoughts together.

64. You can only feel good when you think something that allows you to feel good; you can only feel bad when you think something that allows you to feel bad.

65. What science doesn't understand, it doesn't accept.

66. Choices you make often have nothing to do with what is going on now.

67. How many times do we become what we fear?

68. There's no perfection; it takes 1,000 honest mistakes to master life.

69. If you stay in the moment, you're processing wellness.

70. Energy is the basis of all life.

71. Procrastination is an excuse not to go forward.

72. We don't like to make changes because we don't like how it feels when we're going to lose something.

73. We have too many things in our lives that are superficial and not essential.

74. People who are happy don't have to spend their lives sublimating and escaping to all kinds of other activities.

75. In the presence of happiness, everything else becomes less significant.

76. No one comes to New York City for health. Changing creates health.

77. When people mistrust other people, sometimes it's

because they don't trust themselves.

78. Growth is easy when you have a silent mind.
79. What empowers is the respect you give yourself.
80. We have to disconnect from the non-essential to reconnect to what is essential.
81. Do not be distracted by others' goals.
82. We have a constant need to have a certain image. Why?
83. We have become an achievement-oriented society. In the past thirty years, there were over five million baby-boomer millionaires. Now there are almost one million new baby-boomer millionaires each year. Their whole emphasis is upon the idea that the more I have and the more I own and the more I accomplish and the more I achieve, the more someone is going to respect who I am.
84. Our impermanence scares us.
85. We want everything good to last. We hate loss. This is one source of suffering.
86. You cannot do anything until you engage energy. Engaging the energy precipitates the crisis that leads to change, which brings health.
87. My life works because I make it work. If my life doesn't work, it's because I make it not work. If I go into a championship race, I cannot expect to win if I have not trained as a champion.
88. Trust that everything you need to express and everything you need to communicate is already in place. All you have to do is get out of the way and allow it to express itself.
89. Any time you act opposite to how you naturally are, you won't be fulfilled in whatever it is you are doing. That's why dynamic people should not work for anyone else. Be who you are!

90. Emotions cannot occur unless there is a thought. You create a thought, your thought has an image, the image creates an emotion, and the emotion creates your reaction.

91. We don't know how to rest. When was the last time you spent a day without telephone, beepers, radio, T.V., or talking?

92. Strip us all naked and take away our titles and we're just human beings. It doesn't matter if we're Jewish, Catholic, Black, rich, or poor. Cut us and we all bleed the same red blood.

93. We are not so uniquely different from one another; we pretend to be because that's how we get our image. [may appear to conflict with #49, but does not]

94. Go in and embrace your biggest fears. You'll see that fear is mainly an illusion.

95. Think of how many passages you've been through in life. You have the right to change course; you can go on a hundred paths if you wish.

96. Most of the things we fear losing are imprisoning us.

97. What is the root of envy and jealousy? Is it real or perceived? It is pain from the past, such as sibling rivalry, insidiously triggering pain in the present where there is no real cause for pain.

98. If you're my friend, I don't care what you are. I just care that you're a good person. I like you as a friend. If you're in trouble, I'm going to help you. If you fall down, I'm going to kneel down and pick you up. That's what friends do.

100. Here's the rule: Anyone who is going to gossip to you is going to gossip about you.

101. I'd rather live in a one-room apartment and have unconditional time with the one I love than live in a mansion with a stranger.

102. You pay a price for success. The smart person says no to opportunity once in a while.

103. Do you dissipate energy by doing too much and not doing anything completely?

104. What you want to change may not be what you really need to change. To change what you need to change takes honesty and the courage to sacrifice old habits.

105. Procrastination restricts energy. Action liberates it. Either way you are going to feel energy; one's depleted, one's enhanced. Which do you want?

106. We are on automatic selection instead of making current choices.

107. It's worth going through temporary discomfort to get a health benefit.

108. When we look in the mirror, we should look at what we ideally want to see. Every time you look in the mirror you should see that ideal body. If you don't see the ideal body and all you see is what you have, then you're going to be limited by the vision of what you have as being all that you're capable of having.

109. "Hard" to me is holding onto something that doesn't work, having given it a fair chance.

110. Look for the reasons why you should do what you want to do. Encourage yourself to take action.

111. Don't look for someone or something to change your life. Rescue yourself! Read Emerson's essay on "Self-Reliance."

112. How can you trust someone who is egocentric, powerful, and self-centered? You need to have confidence in yourself, love yourself, and find understanding and balance in life to achieve independence. No one's power should exceed your own. You need to be the strongest person in

your life.

113. We inevitably do this—compare friends, lovers, achievements, and experiences, but this dishonors the present circumstances. Accept where you are in the present moment and be happy.

114. Visualize your achievements and focus your energy and passion—then move fearlessly toward accomplishing your goals. Forget the expectations of others, and your conditioning. Take chances; don't be afraid of others' opinions of you. Be creative and work toward your life.

115. What we give up is important in that we're able to relinquish fears and limitations and gain new understanding and possibilities of feelings, creativity, etc.

116. Do this daily: Don't compromise the essential self and negate that value. Appreciate self in spite of others. Often, you are the only person who'll stand up for you. Be who you are. Don't be afraid of taking a chance to be you, by staying "safe" and predictable.

117. Every painful experience strengthens you for the next one.

118. Remember: growth may threaten others; they don't want a challenge to negate themselves. So, don't look to others for self-validation. You have to validate you.

119. Desire and motivation are keys to accomplishment. You can find ways to use the inherent crises in life as tools to help you grow. If you think you have insurmountable problems and you need inspiration, read *The Story of My Life* by Helen Keller.

120. Eliminate the words "but" and "can't" from your vocabulary and from your life. They will limit and restrict you. Without those words, you can accomplish your goals. Prepare to succeed. Don't allow yourself or others to restrict your progress.

121. Don't impose artificial limits on yourself; discard them.
122. What I want from you in a relationship is quality companionship, honest and open and vivacious, and dynamic conversation with commitment to an ideal or standard of sharing that never abuses trust.
123. Are you ready for what you want?
124. We cannot do something negative and harmful, and then seek a spiritual answer. Does the word "hypocrite" spring readily to mind? How about "sneaky?"
125. You have to do what you want to connect to.
126. No more negative talk.
127. See the ideal that you want to be.
128. Do not mirror anything that makes you feel bad about who you are.
129. You can only care about what you are connected to.
130. When you make the right connection, you do not have to prove anything.
131. Until you can rebel against your complacency, you cannot change.
132. What value did this day have?
133. When you stop fearing change, anything is possible.
134. Stop living at the lowest end of everything.
135. Think of all the (lawful) things you have not done because your beliefs would not allow it.
136. Withdraw from deception and reconnect with honesty.
137. We rarely listen to the person with whom we are in conflict.
138. How can you expand your consciousness if you do not first expand your ideals?
139. Seek what has not yet been discovered; be willing to search for answers that have not yet been found.
140. How many times have you resisted a challenge because

you do not like the idea of being challenged?

141. Identify where you drifted away from your own dreams.

142. Recognize opportunity, don't recognize failure. If someone says, "It's a failure," you see it as an opportunity. Put this thought into your program for growth.

143. Lighten up, loosen up, unwind, and put down your defense mechanisms.

144. If you can't be healthy and whole as an autonomous single, then you'll never be happy in a relationship.

145. Start realizing that what you fear and avoid are what you are. By welcoming new activities, keeping your focus, and taking one more step every day, at the end of a week, your old self recedes, and your new self appears. Get beyond procrastination because in a year from now if you continue to procrastinate, your health will be worse, your mind will be down, your spirit will be broken and life will be beyond you!

146. Take a look at your life. Is it integrated? It must be integrated to be in harmony. Anything that creates disharmony creates conflict; anything that creates conflict creates crisis.

147. Closure is so important in life.

148. Think integral!

149. Be like a bird. A bird never contemplates its own death while it's flying. They don't think of themselves falling out of the sky.

150. Think of a career that would allow you to do the things that fit your life energy.

151. Network your life energy. Partner with someone who will complement your life energy.

152. When you discover what you should be doing, it will be a

revelation. You will not have to work on it or sell yourself
into it. If you have to sell yourself into it, it's not for you.

153. You can only have happy positive feelings if you have
happy positive thoughts.

154. Know that your attitude will change your life!

155. There is nothing more damaging than a mind that is
overly critical of itself and/or of others.

156. Stop over-reacting to everything. Use reason.

157. I have to change me, not the circumstances of my life.

158. Health simplifies life.

159. We must choose to change or we will be forced by some
outside force to change. We must be in control of the
change.

160. Do not allow your pain or disease to become more important than you are.

161. The only people you are able to help are those with you in
that moment.

162. My life should have quality and meaning beyond my
work.

163. Do you blame and complain—or change?

164. We overvalue our possessions and undervalue ourselves.

165. What is so important in the goal that you lose everything
in achieving it?

166. Nothing in life is predictable except complacency

167. You do not need anyone else to make you complete or
whole.

168. Knowledge is both the most important quality to gain and
to surrender. Don't always look for new knowledge, but
rather, seek a new meaning.

169. Most people live predictable lives. There is no potential in
predictable patterns. The world is constantly changing; so

should we. The only time people change is when they are in crisis or when there are no other options, e.g. pioneers. To accomplish changes:

a) People should find a good support system from people who have excelled in their accomplishments;

b) be in the moment; that's when you are most able to change. The moment cannot exist if you control it. We are never free until we disengage the mind;

c) changes should be radical, not small;

d) life should be constantly challenging;

e) nothing ever changes unless we confront it;

f) look for the hero

170. We are born perfect and we spend the rest of our lives denying it.

171. If you don't try to create an image to please other people, then you are able to create a life that's based upon what you really want.

172. When we are rigid in our comforts and standards, we become inflexible.

173. You must look beyond your limitations to be able to transcend a problem. Instead of paying attention to what doesn't work, pay attention to what works. Do not criticize yourself; it's a growth process. Failure doesn't exist if you are being yourself.

174. You will always get what you fear the most. Fear should not dictate what you will or will not do.

175. Winning is not important, it's merely a by-product of attaining excellence.

176. Euphoria and bliss can only occur when the conscious mind has been suspended, surrendered to the moment. It happens to us when we interact with nature and animals.

177. Writing down what's meaningful in your life and picturing where you want to be is an important part of the changing process.

178. The more time you spend with someone, the more you see that part of him that's hidden. We need to have more time to ourselves, rather than spend every minute with another person. Allow more personal space.

179. How many times have you made decisions based on your need to control everything, and based on your discomfort when you can't control things?

180. What we cannot control, we generally destroy. We marginalize.

181. And needing to control a relationship, an environment, a people, a moment, mans that there's not a free flow of energy.

182. What do we do to control the uncertainty of our lives? We try to make things certain. And how do we make things certain? We try to make them permanent.

183. Love is not something someone can give you. Love is something that you feel, and you express it by how you live.

184. It's only when you're vulnerable that you grow, because you are giving yourself the freedom to make errors and be happy with your errors. And you better learn to be happy with the mistakes you make, because if you are angry at the mistakes you make, then you create a self-loathing.

185. Only the quiet mind can heal.

186. And stop trying to figure everything out. Life was never meant to be figured out, it was meant to be lived. There is a big difference.

187. You can either adapt to a situation, or transcend bound-

aries.

188. Stress is not an external happening. Change your reaction and you change the outcome of the stress.

189. Being skilled and successful are not enough after all.

190. Every day, include small optimistic, joyful events. Break your daily ritual. That's one way we can change how we deal with stress because we're now going to make every day a ritual of happiness. Play with a pet, grow flowers, listen to music, prepare a dish to eat or write to a friend.

191. How is fear used to control us?

192. So we look for the medications that keep us comfortable in our suffering.

193. What would you do if fear were not an option?

194. If you need someone to love you to validate you, then it's not love you're seeking, it's validation. Don't call it love. It's need.

195. Are you going to waste a lot of your time trying to be complete through someone else?

196. What you do not address and what you do not change and what you do not reconcile in yourself, you take into a relationship, and now all you have is the incompleteness of two needy people coming together, even if your needs are similar. And all you still have is the insecurity and the stress of knowing you're still incomplete, but in that relationship you are going to try to disguise your incompleteness for fear of having the other person recognize it.

197. Instead of love, we have desire coupled with need, and then we bond with someone superficially and we wrap it in emotion and schmaltz and sexual obligation and all forms of commitments and the first time that is stressed, it breaks.

198. So people over and over again keep taking this incomplete connection and gluing it together. Challenge your relationship, challenge anything in your life you feel is inessential and see whether or not you withstand the challenge and are stronger because of it.

199. I'm suggesting to look at your truths one at a time. Analyze them and say, "Is this truth a universal one?" Could this apply to everyone? And if it can't, then surrender it.

200. Do you only accept information that supports your viewpoints? Do you ignore everything else?

201. That is how we manifest disease—not honoring who we really are and not honoring our core values.

202. Adaptation keeps you in the circle of the known. Transformation transcends the known. Transformation is where the healing is—not in adaptation.

203. Choose a project that forces you to test your beliefs.

204. When we no longer carry blame and shame then self-love evolves. Stop criticizing.

205. When we are accountable on a daily basis for our basic and essential needs, then we prevent conflict.

206. How do you validate what is accurate or distorted? How do you know that what you believe in is real?

207. Are you motivated by outside pressures to do something? Why do you do what you do? And who or what causes you to do it?

208. Do you function from conscious choice (meaning making proper decisions about your life) or fear (or by default)?

209. Education provides tools and rituals, but no spiritual context in which to use them.

210. Fear equals anger. Anger equals unhappiness. Unhappiness equals resentment. Resentment equals greed. Greed

equals obsession and the need to dominate. And that all equals violence. So if you want to look at the extension of violence, go back to what precedes it. Don't just look at the final act. Look at everything that came before it. It's all part of it.

211. We either fear doing something or remember what we did and didn't like. So you shouldn't be caught in the past and you shouldn't be projecting your fear into the future. Life is the moment. Wisdom transcends knowledge in the capacity to function and make proper choices.

212. How often do you remind yourself of past mistakes?

213. Change the word mistake to an experience.

214. I will continue to learn because I'm not afraid to make mistakes.

215. Do you hide from conflict? Do you try to please others?

216. Which rules do you use to prevent risk?

217. No risks, no rewards. Little risks, little rewards. Big risks, big rewards. Taking appropriate risks in life challenges who we thought we were and challenges what we didn't think we could do.

218. Only when you believe that you are enough to be complete in your own life without anyone else's input about what you should do, what you should think and what you should be, are you going to start to realize you can start all over again and recreate your values.

219. Every person has the capacity to change. Who you are, what you do, and how you feel are flexible.

220. Start a day only with positive thoughts: I am going to honor my body, mind, heart and spirit.

221. People confuse the idea of being in live with need. The whole idea of relationships is to enhance each other's life, rather than to be dependent on each other.

222. If you can't change something, change a perception of it, so it won't control you.

223. Rediscover your inner child. Every day, bring up the quality of the childhood: innocence, honesty, curiosity, wonderment, creativity, adaptability, forgiveness, happiness, energy, eagerness to learn, spontaneity, trusting others, lack of inhibition, dreaming the impossible, heroism, no self-condemnation, optimism, resourcefulness, playfulness, love.

224. Love yourself unconditionally!

225. What establishes the limits to what you can or are willing to achieve?

226. Ah! Being skilled and successful are not enough after all. List how you've used your skills to create problems for yourself and others.

227. What would you do if fear were not an option?

228. When we no longer carry blame, shame, and self-criticism, then self-love evolves.

229. What do you distort about your view of yourself? What don't you see accurately?

230. How do you validate what is accurate or distorted?

231. How often do you remind yourself of past mistakes?

232. What is the motivation for what you do?

233. What in our lives is too complicated? What is very simple?

234. What role do deadlines, schedules, goals and play have in our days?

235. Do we have excellent achievements, and not so excellent connections to our real needs?

236. Stop doing anything that is not worth doing.

237. Do you obsess on a single issue or do you bring variety to your thoughts?

238. Images are not necessarily reality.
239. What if most of your fears and shortcomings were not real—just wrong projections?
240. You have the right to design your own life.
241. The eye that sees or the ear that hears is first connected to the past self. If anything is remembered as threatening we may automatically reject it, or if something is remembered as acceptable, we are inclined to embrace it.
242. Our fears are disabling. They prevent us from ever testing them. Are they real?
243. If you believe that you are a failure because you didn't do it right—then everyone's expectation of you, including your own will be lowered.
244. We wait for that special something to happen to ignite our interest, to inspire us to action. We whine and complain like spoiled children for something to occur, while we, ourselves, are unwilling to do it.
245. Don't attack or avoid that which could change your reality. *Don't let fear embalm your beliefs!*
246. When we listen non-judgmentally, we hear everything.
247. In order to believe you can be free or do anything, first you must believe in your completeness.
248. The birth of any new idea, self-actualized, means the death of what it is replacing.
249. Life is in constant change. Do we fear the process of that change?
250. Can you expand your consciousness without first expanding your ideas and values?
251. You resist whatever challenges you.
252. To achieve a meaningful and purposeful goal, we should love it.
253. How often do you say exactly what you: (a) Feel; (b)

Believe; (c) Expect; (d) Need?

254. To what do you completely commit yourself?

255. Which questions and issues do we avoid or allow others to answer for us?

256. As we age, what triggers our need for purpose?

257. Don't ask *how*, rather, affirm *when* you will engage in a transformational process.

258. Are our goals more important than our lives?

259. What boundaries have we accepted from others as if they were our own?

260. Do we control through reward, punishment, or unconditional encouragement?

261. When we strive for constant secure happiness, we create stress as each circumstance evolves.

262. Don't accept your imperfection as limitation.

263. All people are passages in our journey. All were meant to assist us.

264. Did you choose change, or were you forced into it?

265. How do you validate your life? For whom do you do it? We are merely an extension of the common value system of others.

266. What if we choose to reinterpret all of our "realities?" What would change?

267. How does conflict ensue from the need to be right?

268. If you were to step back and look at every part of your life, which part represents the real you? Which parts are authentic? What do your choices reveal about you?

269. Every belief will cause corresponding behavior; examine your behavior if you want to know what you think!

270. Are repetitive thoughts or feelings about any limitation only reinforcing them?

271. If you crave something that you don't have and may never

have, how does that influence the present moment?

272. What will loss and change create?

273. We are frequently disappointed because we are not conscious of the moment; instead, we retreat to the past or project into the future. We just want to be somewhere else, feeling and experiencing something else.

274. When you master the every day habit of just being nice, in time it just becomes effortless.

275. Don't expect or even ask for thanks. Do good because you are good.

276. What happens when we compare ourselves to others or allow others to compare themselves to us?

277. Think of the little kindnesses you've received. What do you remember about them?

278. Focus on the deep pain that you have survived and replace it with kindness.

279. How can we escape the circle of being a victim?

280. Do you risk being unhappy by growing and changing yourself?

281. What situations have you placed yourself into that you have regretted, but you did not have the courage to change?

282. Is challenging yourself to be in motion a dare to surrender each moment?

283. Does the birth of any new idea, self-actualized, mean the death of what it is replacing? Is life in constant change? Do we fear the process of that change?

284. Which questions and issues do we avoid or allow others to answer for us?

285. What opportunities does adversity offer?

286. What do you do that really matters?

287. Change is a matter of letting go. What have you let go of?
288. What in our lives is complete?
289. The more you need others, the less you validate yourself. Describe which of your relationships are/were based on "need" that affected your perceptions of your worth and validity.
290. When you transcend, you automatically grow. What have you transcended up to this point? (Include fears, bad habits, destructive jobs and destructive relationships, toxic foods, procrastination, excuses, etc.)
291. What do you overdo?
292. What do we do to prevent ourselves from being loved?
293. What do we do to keep ourselves from being financially secure?
294. List five things you do to prevent yourself from being happy.
295. Let go of what doesn't have meaning in your life any more. What does it include?
296. What illusions of security are you still clinging to? (food, relationships, money, career, pension, daily habits)
297. Compose forgiveness letters:
    a. Make a list of all the people in your life, past and present who hurt you or prevented you from reaching your potential;
    b. Write letters to them sharing what they did and how it affected you and how you feel about it in graphic detail. Don't worry about penmanship, grammar or choice of words. At the end of each letter, write the phrase, "and I forgive you." And sign your name.
    c. Write a letter to yourself, outlining anything you have engaged in that is self-denigrating, self-destructive or counter-productive in your life. Also include anything

you may have done to hurt anyone else. And forgive yourself.

d. Burn the letters.

298. All of our happiness is based upon the pursuit and acceptance of the pleasures of our possessions—from people, to places, to jobs.

299. When you look back on your life, it's all those special and ordinary moments.

300. Our crises always tell us something.

301. Every crisis has its resolution built in and every resolution can prevent its crisis.

302. We are born pure and perfect and we spend the rest of our lives moving away from that perfection.

303. If we start taking off all these masks everyone wears and all the pretense, you are just left with the same little boys and girls in the playground of life.

304. All the time, I see people who are physically sick because they are sick of their lives.

305. When we feel discomfort, what is our first response? What we should say is, "I don't feel good right now, but I'm going to learn from this. This is an experience that I'm not going to want to repeat and the only way I'm not going to repeat it is to learn from it. Gain something from it.

306. Whenever problems are not honestly addressed, they're going to reappear in other forms. So what does that tell us about addressing problems? Go right up to it, and look it right in the eye no matter what it is.

307. Think of what happens when you're no longer afraid of losing anything. What have you got in its place? Everything. You've got freedom!

308. How many people end up wasting a lot of their time trying to go through life achieving things to prove that they're okay?

309. It's not important who doesn't accept you; it's only important who does.

310. Anything you've done that does not bring you inner peace and satisfaction has been a test of your time. You've only got so much time and when it's gone, that's it. There's a day you wake up and you're no longer able to do everything that you could have. The opportunity is not always going to be there and we don't want to live with the anxiety of having missed life because we were too afraid to break the control that others have had. The day that has meaning is the day that you retake your life.

311. It's very easy to keep doing forever what you have been used to doing and can do well—that's protectionism. But what about going into areas you don't know anything about and starting from scratch? That means you've got to study, you have to learn. You have to be a constant learner in life, which means you have to learn other perspectives and other peoples' ideas and you have to see where balance and imbalance exist.

312. When you accept a belief system, you can no longer challenge it. Then you have to accept all that is negative and self-limiting. Most of the problems we have in this world are due to our refusal to be honest about the belief systems that we are honoring with out lives because it would mean we'd have to challenge the values that we were taught.

313. Needing to win shows that without winning, you feel you are a failure. Always look to see what is motivating you. If you need something, then it means without it you're not

going to feel good. Winning is fine as long as you can cooperate, not just compete.

314. Persons who are insecure need to win, or they never try.

315. What would you do in your life if you weren't afraid of failure?

316. Look at problems as a way of transforming yourself.

317. When you need reward and acknowledgment, you are forced to comply.

318. With every single thing that I do, I must value my consciousness because my consciousness is the deeper, more insightful, and always honest self. I was born with it. I didn't create it. It was given to me. It's a gift. We are all given a perfect consciousness. Our consciousness allows us to make the decision to do something that is ethical and right.

319. Something great happens when conscious people start sharing energy. You create a fusion of consciousness and now you have power.

320. When you give 100% and it is not enough, then what does it tell you? You are giving it to the wrong goal. It shows that the people you are giving it to do not respect what you have given them.

321. Remember, every cell in the body, if it's affected by a virus or a bacterium is affected by something greater. The real haling in the cell is the consciousness of the cell. No cell exists without a consciousness—no cell. Tap that consciousness and you tap the healing power.

322. How do we match our real needs? The inner voice lets us know. Break the pattern of behavior. If the pattern of behavior has led to the disease in the environment, then change the environment, and the pattern.

323. Trust should be earned by our actions, not just by our words.

324. The only people to have in your life are people that can be consistent in honesty, decency, trust, and kindness.

325. If you don't have the confidence of the inner self, then you are always going to be looking for feedback and acceptance from others.

326. Don't look to other people to validate you.

327. Think of all the things that would change if you had love in your heart all the time!

328. No matter what, there's still love here, and as long as there's love, there's the capacity to heal.

329. The trouble is that we've never even learned how to use our minds. Using the mind is not worrying about things—that's never achieved anything. Using the mind is not over-concentration, it's not obsessive thoughts, obsessive behavior. It's relaxing and surrendering to that which is most natural. And what's most natural is the curiosity, the wonderment, the joy, the grace, the loving, the innocence, the honesty to explore life.

330. People who are engaged in life don't think about it.

331. When the world gets to where we don't want to deal with it, we retreat into denial.

332. Eighty percent of a person's active day is engaged in fantasy or escapism. That means that eighty percent of the time is devoted to something else instead of constructively living your life. Imagine what would happen if you started to turn that fantasy into reality.

333. If you don't have a commitment to your higher self, then you commit yourself to the lower self. And the lower self is indulgence and distraction.

334. Spirit allows you to face the crisis and still be okay.
335. Change comes when we seek truth above all superficiality.
336. So much energy is put into deception, and into keeping the deception going.
337. That which honors life is true.
338. How are we ever going to communicate with meaning if we are always communicating with partial deception?
339. Make the right choice—the right choice is the honest choice—not the short-term satisfaction.
340. Stress is not an external happening, rather it is our reaction to what we can't control. Change your reaction and you can prevent stress.
341. General George S. Patton said, "If everyone is thinking alike, then somebody isn't thinking."
342. Your conditioning and your fear of losing control of a situation will keep you using one tool over and over again, even when that tool hasn't helped you.
343. Spiritual truth gives you courage.
344. "The man who goes alone can start today; but he who travels with another must wait till the other is ready."—Thoreau, 1854.
345. Stress comes when you force something to work.
346. The mind that creates the problem cannot be the mind that solves the problem; you need a new mind, or you'll be answering new questions with the old answers you were spoonfed.
347. Do you function by conscious choice or by fear? We have discipline but not for what is essential for us. Education provides tools (and rituals) but no spiritual context in which to use them.
348. To look at the extension of violence, go back to what pre-

cedes it. Don't just look at the final act, look at all that came before it. That's all part of it.

349. All of life is transparent!

350. Connect with that whic   s blissful and you will no longer do anything destructive!

351. We want our heroes to fail so we can feel better about not being able to keep our commitments!

352. Explore life as a child would!

353. You are what you do, not what you say you will do.

354. What we see as our opposite, we try to destroy.

355. We don't work for a living, we work for a standard of living.

356. Much of what we do in life is done in order to be accepted by someone.

357. Images rarely match reality.

358. There is no growth within the individual if you never give them standards that they have to meet.

359. We put all our energy into potential, when we should be living in each moment.

360. Once you get powerful and wealthy, you insulate yourself from people being honest with you.

361. You'll never find someone else's bliss.

362. Protecting what you have takes a lot of energy.

363. There is never a lie in the unconscious.

364. Look for the person who honors life.

365. How do we sabotage our own efforts?

366. There are millions of ways to forgive. Life is more important than pain.

367. Experiences are tangential to life.

368. Anyone who knows of a crime and doesn't raise his or her voice against it is as responsible as the person who commits the crime.

369. The whole idea of forgiveness is to allow oneself to go

forward.

370. We were led to believe that anything you do for yourself is narcissistic. Greed, egotism, and self-righteousness are certainly counter-productive. Self-value, self-love is very positive; to have self-esteem without any guilt is a part of rebalancing.

371. The whole idea of change is that you've got to feel uncomfortable. Change is never going to occur unless there's discomfort. We don't want the consequences of feeling discomfort, so we compromise. But compromise weakens us inside because the inner voice knows what's right, and doesn't like to be lied to. On the outside we do one thing, and inside something else is occurring. I want to see that reconciled. I want to see that whatever you're feeling on the inside, that's what you do outside, that whatever your conscience says, that's what your actions show.

372. The people who really care about you for who you are have got to give you your freedom to be who you are. And if that means letting go of some control, then they've got to let go of control

373. We're drawn to anything that looks like it has an answer that we don't have.

374. People who are in the public eye stay the hell away from the public. They don't want you getting too close. If you get too close, you see it all and you see that there's not a whole lot of difference between them and you, except the circumstances of success, which are frequently just images, the illusion that there's something different. The reality is that there isn't.

375. Always be aware that you may be blaming someone else for not being what you need them to be in order for you to

feel good about yourself.

376. The next time someone tries to put you down, simply do not allow that energy to come in. You have to accept someone else's energy before it becomes real. Until you accept it, it is not real.

377. The empty friend contacts you only if they want something. The true friend shares the joy of presence, lets you be who you are, and never betrays you.

378. The empty worker just collects a paycheck, is on automatic pilot, doesn't care what they're doing, blames other people for everything, never takes responsibility for anything, and is always resentful of anyone who works harder or does more, because it reflects upon what they're not doing.

379. You have to do something each day to affirm that that day is going to be a day you're not going to lose. Select an easy goal for the day in the area that you specifically want to change. In the morning, first thing when you get out of bed, sit down and work out a strategy to achieve that goal, whatever it is, every single day, seven days a week. If you don't do that, you're not going to look at the goal; you're going to look over the goal at some projection that seems impossible. Each day, change something that is possible. At the end of the week, you've achieved seven minor goals; at the end of the month 28–31 minor goals; every three months, an intermediate goal; every six months, a major goal, and every year, a life goal. Then you can say, "I've achieved 365 minor goals, 12 important goals, 2 major goals, and one lifetime goal, all in a year, by doing one thing per day." And that's the purpose of the day. Once you achieve the goal, never take a step back.

380. If you haven't been able to challenge your learning expe-

riences, then you're a very conditioned person. You're going to make it really hard for any change to occur in your life.

381. Anything you're doing that you shouldn't be doing is causing disease. It's changing the energy balance in the body.

382. Just accept something or reject it. If it's not right, you simply let it go because it's not right. If it is right, you accept it because it is right. You don't have to justify it.

383. There's a simple rule. I never allow any of my friends to share gossip with me. Ever. Because it's inevitable. If someone's willing to tell you gossip, they're going to gossip about you. Believe that. If someone's going to betray someone else to you, they're going to betray you.

384. We must consider what may result from the choice we are making.

385. You can only control your action. You can never control a reaction. Choose an action, which has a possibility of having a positive reaction.

386. You cannot expect a miracle to replace constructive, positive, systematic, and disciplined change.

387. What is the attention you need from other people? If you need to be the center of attention and need people to focus upon you and to empathize with you, then it is not a healthy form of recognition.

388. Every day we have to realize the storm will pass, and there will be a rainbow on the other side. We permit distractions such as drugs, alcohol, smoking, gambling, compulsive work and chronic relationships to control us so that we do not have to pay attention to being responsible for understanding why we are not complete, and why we do not have a sense of fulfillment.

389. Think of all the times we thought if only we had something else it would make us happy. It never does.

390. It is only when you are vulnerable that you grow. This gives us the freedom to make errors and be happy with our errors. If we are angry at the mistakes we make, we create self-loathing.

391. We should not surrender to imperfection because you will always be giving up. We should choose to raise the standards of our expectations just a little higher than where we are right now. We must stretch intellectually, physically and spiritually to achieve our goals. Not so high so that we miss the mark, imbalance our lives and cause others to feel very uncomfortable with the efforts we are making. Just high enough to say I did it, and it feels good. Do it enough times so that now you have a new level of comfort and ease in the new standards.

392. Stop trying to figure everything out. Life was never meant to be figured out. Life is meant to be lived. There's a big difference. Challenge what does not make sense and you will wake up and say, "It's a great life." You're going to be able to smile.

393. Frequently, what we become is directly related to what we don't want to be.

394. Everything in life is temporary.

395. When you surrender to the urge to be right, then you allow what is right to exist.

396. If you're open to passion, it's an immediate bridge through all the superficiality of our conditioning.

397. They say, "Give us the science, we will change." We give them the science, they don't change.

398. How can you dismiss ten to twenty billion patient experi-

ences?

399. We have assumed that a title equals knowledge. It does not. Hence, I challenge authority, all authority.

400. Why ask a question when you have the answer?

401. When was the last time you talked with anyone who synthesized the concept of life, instead of compartmentalizing it? You think by compartmentalization, not by synergistic reason. Synergy takes the best of things and puts them together; compartmentalization takes the best of all things and separates them into parts so you can no longer identify your starting material.

402. We have multi-national corporations exploiting every single square inch of this planet. In Africa and Asia where massive poverty exists, do you think these major corporations give back one percent of the income they make for proper wells for water, for sustainable agriculture, to create forests again, to create crop land again, to create proper medical facilities, where the people at least have drugs that work against tuberculosis and malaria; not one penny does any of these Fortune 500 companies give, not a nickel!

403. If you see that you're weak, anything that represents weakness in others, you're going to find abhorrent.

404. I don't want a convenience relationship. Do you know how often people stay in relationships where they do not have love?

405. Most of the things we fear losing, we don't need to begin with. What you feel you cannot live without is not nurturing you, it has imprisoned you. When you become imprisoned by your fears and are not making choices that are in your own best interest, how are you going to choose joy?

406. We grew up in a generation where the energy was still connected, where people still said hello when you walked down the street . . . people smiled . . . people were courteous. I remember once a car stalled in the street. I remember that, like everyone on the street, I ran out to help that person. Here, they'd steal the car!

407. Long after we should have given up our allegiance to false ideals, we continue to support them because we don't want to disappoint the people we feel we have to get permission from before we can grow up and think independently.

408. Now how many people are in your mind at any given time controlling what you think?

409. The people that mean the most to you in your life are not there to entertain or educate you, to impress you or dazzle you. They are there because of the sweetness of their dispositions and the kindness of their souls. And that's what you like about them.

410. I'm concerned that not enough of us have learned the art of play. Play is the joy of affirming our right to be alive!

411. There are people in the world who will accept you exactly as you are. You just have to find them.

9

MOOD-ALTERING RECIPES

WHEN people are either anxious or depressed, they may overeat or lose their appetite altogether. Rarely do they eat what is good for them. When they do eat, people generally go for junk foods or comfort foods. That's when the sugar binging and the chocolate and the pizzas become a form of medication.

For healthy recovery, we must realize that the mind is nourished by positive thoughts, the brain by positive nutrients. We now know that such nutrients as phosphytitleserine, acetyl-l-carnitine, gingko biloba, l-carnitine, choline, B12 are all important for proper brain function as is glutathione and essential fatty acids.

When our diet does not contain the nutrients that are the basic building blocks of a healthy body, then we shouldn't be surprised when, at the end of a day, we do not feel better. We are overfed and undernourished, consuming too many calories from protein and fat, and not enough essential nutrients. We are starving for living foods that have a vital life force, foods that cleanse, detoxify, and flood the body with healing phytonutrients.

This chapter is designed to give you the basic tools—juices and solid foods that are tasty, delicious, easy to prepare, and inexpensive. These foods help the body rebalance its chemistry. Frequently that, in and of itself, is enough to give many people a sense of well being. Follow this diet and you are going to lose weight, cleanse, naturally chelate toxic metals, and stop body pollution. Eliminating toxic foods is the first step. Rebuilding the body with good foods is the second.

Following a good diet is not always easy to do and may take conscious effort. I travel throughout the United States when I am on tour. Recently, I was in Denver, Detroit, Pittsburgh, Washington D.C., Atlanta, and Fort Myers, all in five days. Wherever I traveled, the hotel restaurant food was not what I would consider healthy. The average American, whether at home or on the road, is consuming an enormous amount of unhealthy nutrients.

The recipes in this chapter are designed to correct that by getting you on the road to healthy eating. You can also go to your library and get *The Joy of Juicing Cookbook, The International Vegetarian Gourmet Cookbook, The New Vegetarian Cookbook,* and *Vegetarian Cooking for Good Health*. Feel free to substitute items, where necessary. In my early cookbooks, I included dairy, assuming that organic milk would be fine. Today I would replace that with rice milk or soymilk. Historically, I used organic flour. Today I exclude that and instead use spelt, amaranth, quinoa, millet, oat, or brown rice.

I find that people on a wheat-free, dairy-free, sugar-free, caffeine-free diet have more energy and less weight; they begin to feel better and look better. Sometimes that's all that's needed. Add nutrients and exercise and you're on your way.

Squash Blossoms Stuffed with Barley, Herb & Pine Nuts

Serves 4

24 each Squash or Pumpkin Flowers Washed & Stamen Removed
1 cup Cooked Barley
1 med Onion ¼ inch Small Diced
½ clove Garlic Chopped
1 tsp Thyme Chopped
1 tsp Oregano Chopped
2 tsp Parsley Chopped
1 T Safflower Oil
¼ cup Pine Nuts

1. On low, heat oil and cook onions and garlic.
2. Add thyme, oregano, parsley, pinenuts and barley and heat throughout.
3. Open flowers enough to place barley inside and steam flower for 1–2 minutes.

Calamata Olive Ratatouille

Serves 4

1 large Onion 1 inch diced
2 cloves Garlic chopped
1 each Peppers
1 each Egg Plant – Med 1 inch diced
1 each Zucchini 1 inch diced
1 T Safflower Oil
2 each Tomatoes 1 inch diced, juice saved
½ tsp Rosemary chopped
½ tsp Thyme chopped
1 tsp Basil chopped
Salt & Pepper

1. Sauté onion, zucchini, peppers and eggplant in safflower oil on low heat until vegetables are soft.
2. Add tomatoes and simmer for 10 minutes.
3. Add rosemary, thyme, garlic and basil.
4. Season with salt, pepper and serve.

Chef Notes:
This may be served on its own or with fish, tofu or tempeh.

Mushroom Ragout with Walnuts and Prunes

Serves 4

1 cup Shitakes halved with stem removed and washed
1 cup Crimi sliced with stem removed and washed
1 cup White sliced with stem removed and washed
1cup Maitake sliced with stem removed and washed
1 cup Oyster halved with stem removed and washed
2 T Safflower Oil
½ cup Prunes pitted and split
½ cup Walnuts toasted
1 T Tarragon chopped
2 T Walnut Oil
1 medium Onion ½ inch medium diced

1. Sauté' mushrooms and onions in oil on low heat until any moisture has evaporated. This should take about ten minutes.
2. Add walnuts, prunes, tarragon, garlic and walnut oil.
3. Season with pepper and serve hot or cold.

Chef Notes:
You may use any combination of the above mushrooms or any other mushrooms. The objective is to include as many different mushrooms as possible.

Bass with Fennel, Turmeric and Cumin Coulis

Serves

4 ea 6oz Stripped Bass Filets
2 ea lemons juiced
¼ cup organic white wine

FOR THE COULIS
2 cups Vegetable Stock
1 tsp Turmeric
½ tsp Cumin seeds
2 heads Fennel bulb quartered, cored and 1 inch large diced
1 tsp Tarragon chopped

PREPARE COULIS
1. Put stock, fennel, cumin and turmeric in sauce pan and simmer until fennel is tender.
2. Place this mixture in blender and blend until smooth.
3. Serve coulis with bass.
4. Bake bass with lemon juice and wine on 350° for 10 to 15 minutes.

Chef Notes:
Coulis is term applied to puréed sauces.

Roasted Fall Root Vegetables

Serves 4

1 medium Carrot, not peeled washed and quartered
1 medium Parsnip washed and quartered and core removed
12 each Pearl Onions peeled
12 each Small Heirloom Potatoes
    Russian Fingerlings, German Butterball, Ozette, Yukon, Purple or
    Red Potatoes
4 each Shallots peeled
4 cloves Garlic peeled
1 small Celery Root peeled, 1 inch large dice

¼ cup Balsamic Vinegar
¼ cup Maple Syrup
1 tsp Thyme
½ tsp Coarse Black Pepper

1. Bake vegetables in a pan at 300° for 30–45 minutes, make
   sure potatoes are cooked.
2. Place in a bowl and toss with maple syrup, balsamic
   vinegar, thyme and black pepper.
3. Return to pan and bake for 10 more minutes.
4. Remove and serve.

Marinated Cauliflower and Onions in Curry

Serves 4

1 head Cauliflower core removed and cut into florets
1 medium Onion peeled and ½ inch sliced
2 cloves Garlic peeled whole
2 tsp Madras Curry Powder

¼ cup Apple Cider Vinegar
¼ cup Rice Syrup
½ cup Water
2 each Bay Leaves

1. Bring vinegar, rice syrup, water and bay leaves to simmer.
2. Add curry, garlic, onion and cauliflower, simmer with lid on for 2 minutes.
3. Remove from heat, let cool in liquid at room temperature.
4. After 1 hour place in refrigerator and serve chilled.

Chef Notes:

You may substitute carrots for the cauliflower or your favorite vegetable. I happen to enjoy the flavor the curry combines with cauliflower.

Sardines with Marinated Chickpeas

Serves 4

1 ½ # Fresh Sardine Filets
2 cup Chickpeas cooked
1 each Bell Pepper ½ inch medium diced
1 small Red Onion ½ inch medium diced
2 T Chives sliced thin
¼ cup Sunflower Seeds
4 each Lemons juiced
1 tsp Cumin Seeds
½ cup Extra Virgin Olive Oil
1T Flax Oil
1 T Parsley

1. Bake sardine filets for 8–10 minutes at 350°.
2. Mix the remaining ingredients.
3. Pour chickpeas on top of sardines and let marinate for 4 hours.
4. Serve chilled.

Cod with Mustard and Garlic

Serves 4

4 6oz Cod Filets
½ cup Dijon Mustard
2 cloves Garlic chopped
1 tsp Thyme chopped
1 tsp Rosemary chopped
1 tsp Tarragon chopped

1. Mix mustard, garlic, thyme, rosemary and tarragon.
2. Apply mustard mixture on cod fillets and bake at 350° for 10–12 minutes.

Chef Notes:
This is a very simple recipe that also works well with salmon.

Bass with Kalamata Olives, Tomatoes and Garlic

Serves 4

4 6oz Sea Bass Filets

½ cup Kalamata Olives pitted
2 each Garlic Cloves chopped
1 large Tomato 1 inch large diced with juice
1 cup Organic White Wine
2 T Basil lightly chopped
1 T Parsley lightly chopped
2 T Extra Virgin Olive Oil

1. Place Bass and olives, garlic, tomatoes and wine in a covered baking dish and bake at 350° for 20 minutes.
2. Remove from oven when fish is cooked and top with basil, parsley and oil.

Chef Notes:
Herbs should always be chopped lightly. Over chopping herbs will alter the taste of them. Using a sharp knife is equally as important. These two step will help keep the fresh vibrant flavor of herbs.

Tilapia with Mango-Ginger Salsa

Serves

4 each 6 oz Tiapia Filets
Canola or Safflower Spray

FOR THE MANGO-GINGER SALSA
½ cup Mango or Pineapple Juice fresh squeezed
2 each Mangos ½ inch medium diced
1 med Red Onion ½ inch medium diced
½ each Green Pepper ½ inch medium diced
½ each Red Pepper ½ inch medium diced
1 T Ginger chopped
1 T Cilantro lightly chopped
1 T Basil lightly chopped
2 each Scallions sliced

1. Heat a Teflon sauté pan on medium heat and lightly spray tilapia with canola spray.
2. Sauté tilapia until brown on low heat.
3. Mix all ingredients of salsa and serve cold or warm with fish.

Chef Notes:

This salsa may be served on its own as light lunch or with some brown rice for a heavier meal.

Alaskan Halibut with Braised Fennel

Serves 4

4 ea 6 oz Alaskan Halibut Filets

2 heads Fennel Bulb cored and split in 6 wedges
2 cups Vegetable Stock
1 tsp Fennel Seed
$\frac{1}{2}$+ cup Organic White Wine
1 tsp Tarragon lightly chopped
2 ea lemons juiced

1. Place fennel, vegetable stock, fennel seed, wine and tarragon in Corning baking dish with lid and bake at 350° for 1 hour until fennel bulbs are soft.
2. Place halibut filets with fennel and bake for additional 15 minutes at 350° with lid on.
3. Drizzle lemon juice on fish and serve.

Trout Baked in a Fennel Ginger Coulis

Serves 4

4 each Boneless Trout Filets

FOR THE COULIS
1 large Fennel head core removed and dice
1 T Ginger chopped
1 medium Onion ½ inch medium diced
1 cup Vegetable Stock
¼ cup Organic White Wine
¼ tsp Fennel Seed

1. Place stock, fennel, ginger, onion, wine and fennel seed in a covered sauce pan and simmer for 10 minutes until fennel is soft.
2. Let mixture cool for 20–30 minutes and then puree in blender.
3. Pour mixture on top of trout in a ceramic baking dish with lid and bake for 15–20 minutes at 375°.

Salmon Poached in Ginger Broth with Onions

Serves 4

4 each 6 oz Wild Salmon Filet
2 each Garlic Cloves crushed
1T Ginger chopped
4 oz Organic White Wine
2 each Lemons juiced
½ cup Water purified
1 T Braggs Liquid Aminos
2 each Medium Onions ¼ inch sliced

1. Place salmon in a Corning baking dish with lid and add all other ingredients.
2. Place lid on and bake for 25 minutes at 350°.

Chef Notes:
Wild Alaskan Salmon is available fresh from May to October; otherwise some health food stores carry a frozen product for out of season. Wild Salmon has a higher concentration of the heart healthy fats than farmed Atlantic Salmon.

Steamed Purple Potatoes with Basil

Serves 4

2 lbs. Purple Potatoes washed

2 cups Whole Basil Leaves
1/3 cup Extra Virgin Olive Oil
Cracked Black Pepper

1. Boil or steam potatoes until cooked but firm. Cut potatoes in half.
2. Place oil and basil in a blender and puree being careful not to over blend.
3. Toss potatoes with basil oil and sprinkle with black pepper.

Chef Notes:
This is a very simple, but flavorful, recipe. Use the freshest basil possible since it is the highlight of the dish.

Green Tea and Tamari with Bok Choy

Serves

3 tea bags Green Tea
2 cups Water
1 T Lemon Grass chopped
1 clove Garlic crushed
¼ cup Lite Tamari

1 head Bok Choy washed and sliced
1 T Toasted Sesame Oil

1. Bring water to boil and add tea, lemon grass and garlic.
2. Steep for 5 minutes, then remove tea bag.
3. Return mixture to a boil, add tamari and bok choy.
4. Cook bok choy until it just starts to soften.
5. Serve hot with tamari-tea and drizzle sesame oil on bok choy.

Chef Notes:
Feel free to add other vegetables such as onions or broccoli.

Barley and Pearl Onions with Honey, Mustard and Tahini Dressing

Serves 4

DRESSING
2 T Honey
2 T Tahini
2 T Dijon Mustard
2 T Apple Cider Vinegar
½ cup Safflower Oil
¼ cup Raw Apple Cider Vinegar
1 tsp Thyme chopped
2 cups Barley cooked
16 each Pearl Onions peeled

1. Place onions in four cups of cold water. Bring to a simmer on medium-low heat. Simmer onions until tender. Strain and cool onions.
2. Add honey, tahini, mustard and vinegar to a blender.
3. While blending drizzle oil in to make a creamy dressing.
4. Mix dressing to barley, onions and thyme and serve chilled.

Apple Jicama and Cumin Salad

Serves 4

2 each Apples-Granny Smith cored and ½ inch diced with skin
1 med Jicama skinned and ½ inch diced
1 tsp Cumin Ground
3 ea Scallions chopped lightly
1 ea Red Pepper ½ inch diced
1 T Mint chopped lightly
⅓ cup Basic Vinaigrette
¼ tsp Turmeric

1. Mix all ingredients and serve.

Chef Notes:

Use a small electric coffee grinder to grind spices. Cumin, fennel seed, coriander, allspice, cinnamon and any other spices work well.

Celeriac and Orange Salad

Serves 4

2 cups Celeriac Root peeled and ½ diced
3 each Scallions sliced
2 each Oranges juiced
¼ tsp Ground Cardamom
¼ tsp Course Ground Black Pepper
1 T Mint lightly chopped
2 each Oranges peeled and sliced
⅓ cup Basic Vinaigrette

1. Mix All ingredients in a bowl and serve.

Bulgur-Pine Nut, Pumpkin Seed, Sunflower Seed, Mint and Cucumber

Serves 4

1 cup Bulgur Wheat cooked
⅓ cup Boiling Water
2 T Lemon Juice
2 T Extra Virgin Olive Oil
2 T Pine Nuts
1 T Sunflower Seeds hulled-raw
1 T Pumpkin Seeds hulled-raw
1 medium Cucumber ½ inch diced
2 tsp Mint chopped
2 tsp Parsley chopped

1. Mix all ingredients together and serve.

Basic Vinaigrette

½ cup Apple Cider Vinegar
2 T Dijon Mustard
1 T Tahini
1 T Honey
2 cloves Garlic peeled
1 cup Expeller Pressed Sunflower Oil
¼ cup Extra Virgin Olive Oil
½ cup Walnut Oil
2 T Flax Oil
1 T Parsley lightly chopped
1 tsp Thyme lightly chopped
1 tsp Rosemary lightly chopped
Pepper, white ground

1. Blend vinegar, mustard, tahini, honey and garlic in a blender.
2. While blender slowly drizzle all the oils in. This will cause the vinaigrette to become creamy.
3. After all the oil has been incorporated add the thyme, rosemary and parsley. Season with white pepper to taste.

Super Healthy Vinaigrette

Make the basic vinaigrette but add the following ingredients at the end.

10 to 20 drops Pau D'arco tincture alcohol free
10 to 20 drops Milk Thistle tincture alcohol free
10 to 20 drops Burdock tincture alcohol free
10 to 20 drops Ginseng tincture alcohol free
2–4 drops essential Oil of Oregano
2–4 drops essential Oil of Rosemary
2–4 drops essential Oil of Thyme
2–4 drops essential Oil of Basil

Add one or all of these ingredients for added health benefits.

Mushroom Salad with Burdock Vinaigrette

2 T Safflower Oil
1 cup Shitakes stemmed ¼'d and washed
1 cup White Mushrooms sliced, stemmed and washed
1 cup Portabellos stemmed, gills removed, sliced and washed
1 large Onion medium ½ inch diced
1 clove Garlic chopped
1 stalk Burdock – whole
½ cup Basic Vinaigrette
20 drops Burdock tincture

1. Cook all mushrooms in sauté pan with oil on low. Cook until mushrooms are soft and any excess water has evaporated and let cool.
2. Wash and scrub Burdock, then grate of thinly slice.
3. Add to mushrooms to basic vinaigrette with burdock tincture. Serve warm or cold. It is best to let marinate for 4 to 36 hours.

Curried Lentils

Serves 4

1 cup French Lentils sorted and rinsed
2 tsp Curry Powder
1 tsp Safflower Oil
1 med Onion ¼ inch small diced
¼ cup Raisins
2 each Apples ¼ inch small diced
1 T Apple Cider Vinegar
3 T non-toasted Sesame Oil
1 tsp Basil lightly chopped

1. Bring 6 cups of water to a boil, add lentils and boil for 25 minutes until lentils are firm but cooked, drain them and rinse under cold water.
2. Toast curry powder in a pan in the oven at 350 for 5 minutes.
3. Add safflower oil to a sauté pan and gently cook onions until soft. After the onions are cooked add them to the lentils along with curry, raisins, apples, vinegar, coconut oil and basil.

Kombu Noodle with Sesame

Serves 4

8 oz Kombu Noodles thawed
½ cup Pepper ½ inch medium diced
¼ cup Red Onions ½ inch medium diced
3 each Scallions sliced
1 tsp Ginger chopped
1 tsp Sesame Seeds
2 T Braggs Liquid Aminos
2 T Toasted Sesame Oil

1. Mix all ingredients and serve.

Chefs Note:
Kombu Noodles can be purchased in Health or Oriental food stores frozen section.

Corn, Fennel and Murshooms

Serves 4

1 cup Frozen Corn Kernels thawed-cooked and cooled
2 each Fennel Bulb thinly sliced, core removed
8 oz White Mushrooms stemmed, washed, cooked and cooled
8 oz Shitake Mushrooms stemmed and washed, cooked and cooled
½ cup Basic or Super Healthy Vinaigrette
1 T Tarragon chopped lightly
1 tsp Thyme chopped
1 tsp parsley-chopped lightly

1. Mix all ingredients together and serve.

Soybeans with Green Onions and Sesame

Serves 4

4 cups Soybeans, fresh or frozen cooked and cooled
6 each Scallions sliced
2 T Sesame Oil
1 tsp Mint lightly chopped
1 T Braggs Liquid Aminos
2 tsp Lemon Juice
2 T Sesame Seeds
1 clove Garlic chopped
1 tsp Dulse Flakes

1. Combine all ingredients and serve chilled.

Potato and Nettle Salad

Serves 4

2 lbs Yukon Potatoes 1 inch cubed
3 each Scallions sliced
2 cups Nettle Leaves washed

½ cup Basic Vinaigrette
1. Cook potatoes by placing them in cold water and bring them to a simmer. Cook potatoes for about 15–20 minutes. Check potatoes with paring knife to test for doneness.
2. Cool the potatoes in cold water and drain.
3. Bring 1 pint of water to boil and cook nettles for 5 seconds
4. Strain nettles and cool in an ice water bath. Next chop nettles lightly.
5. Mix all ingredients in a bowl and serve.

Heirloom Tomatoes

Serves 4

4–8 each Heirloom Tomatoes sliced
1 T Basil lightly chopped
¼ cup Extra Virgin Olive Oil

1. Slice tomatoes and line them on an oversized plate, top
   with basil and olive oil.

Chef Notes:
This dish works best when tomatoes are in season in your geo-
graphic area. Sleets tomatoes that are ripe a full of flavor. Most
tomatoes will work, but any heirloom variety is preferred. Do
not be discoursed by the appearance of heirloom tomatoes,
they are usually full of flavor.

Never refrigerate a tomato, room temperature tomatoes taste
and store better.

3 Bean and Oregano Salad

Serves 4

½ cup Kidney Beans cooked
1 cup White Beans cooked
½ cup Anasazi Beans cooked
½ cup Basic Vinaigrette
2 T Oregano lightly chopped
1 clove Garlic peeled and chopped

1. Mix all ingredients. This dish can be saved for up to three days.

Chef Notes:
Any beans will work, even the addition of a fresh green bean.

Purslane and White Bean

Serves 4

2 cup White Beans cooked
1 cup Purslane Leaves washed
2 cloves Garlic chopped
1 tsp Rosemary chopped
1 T Basil lightly chopped
1 T Parsley, Italian lightly chopped
¼ tsp Black Pepper coarsely grounds
1 T Balsamic Vinegar
1 T Apple Cider Vinegar
¼ cup Sunflower Oil
¼ cup Extra Virgin Olive Oil

1. Mix all ingredients and serve chilled.

Bean Cassoulet with Herb Sprout Crumbs

Serves 4

1 T Safflower
2 med Onions ¼ inch diced
2 cloves Garlic chopped
1 each Green Bell Pepper ¼ inch diced
1 cup White Beans cooked
1 cup Kidney Beans cooked
1 cup Garbanzo Beans cooked
1 large Tomato diced
1 tsp Thyme chopped
1 tsp Basil lightly chopped
1 tsp Rosemary chopped
1 tsp Parsley lightly chopped

3 slices Fresh Sprout Bread
3 T Extra Virgin Olive Oil

1. Heat safflower oil on low in sauté pan and cook onions, peppers and garlic gently until soft. Add beans, tomato, ¾ teaspoon of thyme, ¾ teaspoon basil, and ¾ teaspoon rosemary. Heat thoroughly.
2. Place bean mixture in casserole dish.
3. Take bread and puree in food processor with rest of herbs and 1 tablespoon of olive oil.
4. Top beans with bread crumbs and bake at 375° for 20 minutes until bread curbs are toasted.
5. Remove and drizzle with remaining olive oil.

Potato Nettle Soup

Serves 4

1# Yukon Potatoes ½ and washed
3 cups Vegetable Stock
½ med Onion chopped
2 cups Nettle Leaves washed

1. Slow simmer potatoes and onions in vegetable stock until cooked.
2. Add nettle leaves and cook for one minute.
3. Place in blender and puree until smooth.

Miso with Lettuce Soup

Serves

1 medium Onion ¼ inch small diced
1 clove Garlic chopped
1# Tofu-firm ½ inch medium diced
6 cups Vegetable Stock
2 tsp Ginger chopped

to taste Mixed Seaweed
   Hijiki, Kombu, Kelp, Nori

3 each Scallions sliced
1 T Cilantro lightly chopped
1 T Basil lightly chopped
1 T Mint lightly chopped
1 T White Miso
3 cups Greens: sliced very thinly
   Romaine, Spinach, Iceberg, Red Leaf, Chard

1. Simmer onion, garlic, tofu, ginger and seaweed in vegetable stock for 5 minutes.
2. Add miso, scallions, cilantro, basil, mint, and greens and serve.

Chef Notes:

Never simmer miso, so always add miso to a recipe after the cooking process is done. There are several types of miso available, experiment and use the one you like the best.

Potato, Corn and Cashew Soup

Serves 4

1 # Yukon Potatoes halved and washed
5 cups Vegetable Stock
½ cup Cashews- unsalted soaked in water over night
1 med Onion diced
1 clove Garlic peeled

1 cup Soy Milk
½ tsp Thyme chopped
½ cup Corn Kernels cooked

1. Cook potatoes, onions, cashews and garlic in stock until tender. This should take around 30 minutes. Add soy milk and thyme.
2. In a blender purée until smooth.
3. Add corn and return to simmer for one minute.

Chef Notes:
Always choose the smallest possible potatoes available. Pound for pound smaller potatoes have more skin. The skin has a lot of flavor and more concentrated nutrition.

Mushroom and Miso Soup

Serves 4

1 medium Onion ½ inch medium diced
1 clove Garlic chopped
2 cups Mixed Mushrooms washed and cut into bit size pieces
        Shitake
        Miatake
        Oyster
        Woodear
        White or Brown
6 cups Vegetable Stock
1 T Dark Miso
2 tsp Braggs Liquid Aminos

1 T Dulse Flakes
1 T Basil lightly chopped
2 tsp Cilantro lightly chopped
4 each Scallions sliced

1. Gently simmer onions, garlic and mushrooms in vegetable stock for 8–10 minutes.
2. Add miso, braggs, dulse, basil, cilantro and scallions.
3. Serve.

Chef Notes:
Tofu would make a simple addition.

Puree of Carrot and Fennel Soup

Serves 4

1 bulb Fennel chopped with core removed
2 large Carrots washed and chopped
5 cups Vegetable Stock
1 each Bay Leaf
1 sprig Thyme
½ tsp Fennel Seeds

1 cup Soy Milk or Rice Milk
¼ cup Honey

1. Simmer fennel, carrots, bay leaf, fennel seeds and thyme in vegetable stock until vegetables are tender.
2. Add honey and soy or rice milk and blend until smooth.

Cold Potato Spinach and Nettle Soup

Serves 4

1 lbs Yukon Potatoes washed and halved
1 med Onion diced
4 cups Vegetable Stock
1 clove Garlic peeled

2 cups Spinach washed and loosely packed
2 cups Nettle Leaves washed and loosely packed

2 cups Soy Milk or Rice Milk

1. Cook potatoes, onions and garlic in stock until tender. This should take around 30 minutes.
2. Add spinach and nettles and simmer for two more minutes. Add soy milk and thyme.
3. In a blender purée until smooth.
4. Let soup cool and serve.

Chef Notes:

Always choose the smallest possible potatoes available. Pound for pound smaller potatoes have more skin. The skin has a lot of flavor and more concentrated nutrition.

Left over cooked salmon would make a good addition to this soup.

#44

Vegan French Onion Soup

Serves

6 cups Vegetarian Beef Base/stock
2 large Onions peeled, split and ¼ inch sliced
2 cloves Garlic chopped

4 slices Sprout Bread toasted and cut in ¼'s
4 slices Vegetarian Swiss Cheese

1 tsp Thyme chopped
2 tsp Braggs Aminos

1. Divide onions into thirds, take ⅓ of onions and roast them in an oven at 425° for 20–30 minutes. The onions should turn brown without burning.
2. Bring stock to a boil and add roasted onions, ⅓ more raw onions and simmer for 10 minutes.
3. Add the last ⅓ of onions and turn off.
4. Add Thyme and Aminos.
5. Ladle into oven proof crocks, add bread and cover bread with cheese.
6. Place under broiler until cheese melts and browns, serve immediately.

Buckwheat Soba with Pecans and Vegetables

Serves 2–3

1–7 oz package Soba Noodles cooked according to label

1 cup Pecan Halves or Pieces soaked overnight in 2 cups water
   and ¼ Braggs Aminos

2 cloves Garlic chopped
½ cup Onions 1 inch large diced
½ cup Celery 1 inch large diced
½ cup Carrots 1 inch large diced
1 cup Broccoli Florets
½ cup Shiitake Mushrooms stem removed, washed and sliced
½ cup Chinese Cabbage shredded
½ cup Bell Peppers 1 inch large diced

THE SAUCE
3 T Peanut Butter Natural
1 T Toasted Sesame Oil
1 T Bragg Aminos
½ cup Vegetable Stock
1 T Cilantro

1. Blend all in the ingredients for sauce.
2. Steam onions, celery, carrots, broccoli, shiitakes, cabbage
   and peppers until just cooked.
3. Bring sauce to a simmer and add pecans, soba, garlic and
   vegetables.

Broccoli Rabe with Brown Rice Penne, Garlic and Extra Virgin Olive Oil

Serves

½ lb Brown Rice Penne cooked
½ cup Vegetable Stock
1 bunch Broccoli Rabe washed
1 T Safflower Oil
4 cloves Garlic chopped

3 T Extra Virgin Olive Oil
1 T Parsley lightly chopped
1 T Basil lightly chopped

1. Cook Broccoli Rabe by boiling in water for 1–3 minutes.
2. In a sauté pan add oil and cook garlic on low for ½ minute.
3. Add penne, broccoli rabe and vegetable stock.
4. Serve and drizzle olive oil, parsley and basil.

Tempeh and Kidney Bean Chili

Serves 4

1 T Safflower Oil
½ medium Onion ¼ inch small diced
½ Jalapeño Chile ¼ inch small diced
4 cloves Garlic chopped
½ tsp Cumin
4 T Chili Seasoning no salt and non-irradiated
1 T Tomato Puree
1 cup Dry Kidney Beans soaked overnight in 3 cups of water

1 2–3in Piece of Kelp
4 cups Vegetable Stock Reserve 1 cup for chili

2 T Black strap Molasses

1. Rinse Beans and bring them to a simmer with stock and kelp. Cook beans until tender while holding their shape.
2. In a soup pot on low heat add the oil
3. Gently cook onion, garlic and jalapeño until tender.
4. Add Tempeh, cumin, tomato puree, molasses, chili seasoning and beans.
5. Add vegetable stock if necessary.
6. Cook slowly for 20 minutes and serve.

Pasta e Fagoli

Serves 2–4

½ lb Quinoa Pasta cooked
½ cup White Beans soaked over night in 1 ½ cups water
3 cups Vegetable Stock
1 2–3 inch piece Kelp
½ cup Celery ½ inch medium diced
½ cup Carrots ½ inch medium diced
½ cup Onions ½ inch medium diced
1 sprig Rosemary
1 sprig Thyme
1 each Bay Leaf
4 cloves Garlic crushed

1. Rinse beans after soaking, bring beans and vegetable stock to a simmer. Remove any foam that forms on top during the cooking process.
2. Add kelp, thyme, rosemary, bay leaf, garlic, onions, celery, and carrots. Cook beans until tender while they are still holding their shape.
3. When beans are cooked, add cooked pasta.
4. If beans have absorbed all the stock, simply add more until the desired consistency.

10

TESTIMONIALS

Jacqueline Cox, age 46
Gas was a problem. This has been reduced. Ridges in my nails have disappeared. I have lost weight. The color of my skin has changed and it looks better. I am sleeping more. I am tired at 11:30 each night and am getting more sleep. I have more regular and daily bowel movements. I had some chest pains. They have reduced and I have had only one episode I the past three months. My skin is not as dry and is softer. My sugar cravings have reduced.

Shawn Cox, age 35
I have lost 15 pounds. I have lost the negative mindset that would stop me from achieving my goals. I can see things that I could not see before that are the most important in my life such as spending more time with my family.

Marsha Perry Starkes, age 49
My brain fog is beginning to lift. I am able to see my shortcomings more easily. I am beginning to develop self-motivation especially in exercising. I have lost 6–7 pounds.

Michael Johnson, age 46
My blood pressure went from 180/110 to 150/90. I have dia-

betes and my sugar level was averaging 140–160. Now it is 80–140. I lost 10 pounds. I believe I am more forgiving of myself and others.

Andre Partlow, age 26
When I keep my environment clean and uncluttered my thinking is clearer and I just feel better because it's clean and in order. When I don't eat late I sleep deeper, wake with more energy and need less sleep. I also had changes with my blood work.

Yacine Houari, age 51
I had back pain which has improved. I was overweight and I lost 30 pounds. My lack of stamina had improved and I finished the New York Marathon. My mood has improved and also my skin quality.

Anastasia Koutsouras, age 18
I have lost some weight and body fat. My nails are growing nicely. I don't know if this is related but my sweat doesn't smell as much. I have mild asthma, but I feel that I can breathe easier now. When I go to bed, I fall asleep right away. I used to toss and turn for a long time before I could sleep. I've noticed I have more energy.

Lucyna Sadowska
I needed to lose weight and I lost 4 pounds. My concentration improved and also my clarity of thinking and focus. I learned how to control my emotions.

Halina Baranski, age 56
My fatigue is gone. I have better clarity of mind and better com-

pletion of tasks. My wrinkles are almost gone.

Tamara Baranski, age 35

Before I was not able to trust myself 100% and did not have the will power to quit eggs and cheese. I also had acne. Now I trust myself 200%, I have quit cheese and eggs and my acne is almost gone.

Simone Roberts

I came here specifically for losing weight, hypothyroid and rapid pulse. I am off medication for the hypothyroid and rapid pulse. Instead I took 3 weeks off from work and I feel much better. I am proactive in my medical care, not allowing the doctor to categorize me. The biggest change in me is my mindset. I have tried for the past 3 years to be a positive thinker but with this study it has become a reality. I stop myself from being negative. I also found out that I used to be a blamer. Everything is someone else's fault. Now I am working on looking for the positive, what is to be learned and responding in the positive. Thank you all!

Bobby Whitsett, age 45

I notice my skin has more vigor. I notice an increase I strength at the gym. My eyes don't tire as easily and I recall things more. My body fat has decreased and I have more energy to do thins after work.

Bridget Carles, age 49

I started the protocol April 15, 2002 in Naples, FL. I have lost 25 pounds and reversed arthritis in my right ankle and hips. I no longer need cane. I can power walk 1 hour each day and can dance, jog, play tennis and baseball. Formerly I barely hobbled around. Many liver age spots have vanished and many have now improved texture and are disappearing. My fatigue is gone. I have 3 small kids (under 12 years), work 6 days a week and am never tired anymore. I have a much-improved attitude—joy and positivism. Formerly I lost all desire for marital intimacy (sex) and hated my husband's requirements. Now my libido is off the charts; my responses are as good or better than 20 years ago. The cells of my body are vibrating in a new, fantastic way!

Tom Graham, age 70
I now have my anger completely under control. I am more spiritual now than I have ever been. I now live in harmony with nature. I exercise mow more frequently than I have ever exercised in my life. As a consequence of all of these changes I feel healthier now than ever before.

Francie Smilowitz, age
During the support group I lost over 7 pounds and gained more energy. I have less pain in my body. I created wonderful new relationships which honor the emerging me. I already had chosen wheat free, dairy free diet but sometimes made no time to eat. Now I have regular mealtimes and stay on the dietary protocol. I now have better concentration. I took responsibility for each change and chose to honor alignment of mind, body and spirit so that continually whatever was out of alignment became an awareness to me so I could really make a conscious choice or begin to. I made more time for breath, meditation and energy work. The weekly reminder of being in the support group meeting where I was present with people who had also chosen to honor and take responsibility for their holistic health and life was very positive for me. I now take the time to read more, have begun to restructure my relationships and to express myself more.

Tamarah Cabrera, age 45

My fatigue is gone and I am able to sleep 4–5 hours a night and feel rested and energized. I have more mental clarity and I can do many things at a time successfully. From being mildly depressed I now am able to look at problem solving in a positive way. Formerly I was doing no exercise at all. Now I am power walking 3–5 times a week, doing yoga 3 times a week and have participated in races and even the New York Marathon. I lost 3% body fat. Before I participated in the support group I was not able to make decisions. Now I know I can do whatever I would like to and I have the will to follow through!

Harriette Berman, age 58

Previously I had an inferiority complex and confusion of mind; now I have a stronger sense of self and clarity of mind. My depression has lifter and I do not cry so easily. I am better organized and on time. My messiness has lessened. Instead of eating late at night I now eat much earlier. My dry skin has improved especially my facial skin. I drink much more water now where before I drank none.

Diane Rodriquez, age 50

I have changed my bad eating habits and now eat an organic vegetarian diet. I have much less fatigue but still experience some. I plan to relieve this fatigue by more exercise. I lost 10 pounds. When I was heavier I didn't feel well, couldn't breathe and my upper chest felt heavy. Now I can run and can go up stairs easily.

Carol Allen

I had pain in my knees before but now I can do deep knee bends comfortably. I lost 8 pounds and have increased the distance of my running. I feel I am just getting started.

CONCLUSION

LET'S reflect upon what we've learned. Depression cannot be as easily defined as we've been led to believe. Crises arise in life—losses, fears, insecurities, anticipations, grief—and these can alter our mood. Psychiatry has taken it upon itself to determine that anything that varies from a happy frame of mind can fall into the net of depression. Clearly, there are some people with specific brain chemical imbalances. For those individuals, there are natural and nontoxic remedies available that work equally well but without the side effects of the selective seratonin reuptake inhibitors and other drugs. The vast majority, however, do not fit into this category. Children and seniors, the most vulnerable members of our society, must take special care to stay away from psychiatric manipulation and mass marketing.

Where anxiety and depression do exist, Americans need to pay attention to diet. We eat fast foods—a mind-numbing variety of junk foods, foods laced with colorings and pesticides, and now genetically altered foods. We know that sugars, artificial sweeteners, and allergic molecules of food can trigger brain reactions that manifest as anxiety or depression. Add to that the harmful chemicals we breathe and polluted water we drink and you will get an even larger picture of the problem. We live in a toxic cesspool, and this can adversely affect both body and mind. The degree of contamination is so great, in fact, that scientists have correlated its effects to changes in the DNA of unborn children!

Sadly, we are not being honest about the true causes of our dilemma. To do so would be to reveal the corporatization of American culture, where what is good for big business is good for America. Our reaction is, in effect, rather schizophrenic. On one hand we have the Surgeon General, the U.S. Public Health Service, and the National Institutes of Mental Health coming forward and stating that we should clean up our act by taking fast food operations out of hospitals and schools and replacing them with better quality fare. We will not act on this common sense advice, though, because it would mean eviscerating a $300 billion dollar a year industry. Special interest groups contribute substantial amounts of money and, with it, gain access and influence to politicians.

At the end of the day, truth is not what we're given but manufactured—carefully spun propaganda. We're caught in this paradox. We know the truth but cannot utter it. There are too many people who paid for the lie. When you look at the amount of people who have invested in the disease-producing businesses that give us obesity, heart disease, cancer, arthritis, as well as mood-altering illnesses, you see that they are the most powerful among us. They are not only the Fortune 500 companies, but they have an interlocking board of directors on banks. They include large regimens of scientists, physicians, paid consultants who do their bidding before Congressional hearings and for the major media.

How then does the average person with access to none of the above find the truth and make changes? First, do not wait for the mainstream media. They are, by default, limited in what they can offer. Only the most naïve would still believe that we have a truly free and democratic press. Nor can we count upon the objectivity, reasonableness, and humanity of the medical community. They are too conditioned in their own behavior. We must therefore take it upon ourselves to begin the process of networking, to find health support groups, to find counselors and holistic physicians who can help us identify what may be causing our problems and who can show us sensible ways of eliminating our conditions and rebalancing ourselves.

Millions of Americans are on their own unique journeys of healing. They are moving away from the strictly orthodox point of view and opening themselves up to alternative perspectives. The rest of us would be wise to follow their example. For further information, go to garynull.com; look under mental health and visit our online health support group for depression and anxiety.

APPENDIX FOR ALTERNATIVE HEALTH STUDIES

ACUPUNCTURE AND ELECTROACUPUNCTURE

At Beijing Medical University, two consecutive clinical studies on the treatment of depression with electroacupuncture (EA) were conducted. Results from both studies showed that the therapeutic efficacy of EA was equal to that of amitriptyline for depressive disorders. EA had a better therapeutic effect for anxiety somatization and cognitive process disturbance of depressed patients than amitriptyline, and the side effects were much less. [1]

At the University of Mainz, patients in major depression who experienced acupuncture improved slightly more than patients treated with mianserin alone.[2]

At Exeter Hospital, acupuncture was as effective in treating nausea of pregnancy as a sham procedure.[3]

In Germany, results indicate that needle acupuncture led to a significant clinical improvement as well as to a remarkable reduction in anxiety symptoms in patients with minor depression or with generalized anxiety disorders.[4]

In Minneapolis, alcohol use was assessed, along with depression and anxiety, when treated with acupuncture and significant improvement was shown on nearly all measures.[5]

In Ontario, Canada, acupuncture was shown to alleviate depression in patients receiving opiates for chronic non-malignant pain.[6]

At the University of Exeter, acupuncture was shown to be useful in reducing anxiety in the treatment of cancer patients.[7]

At Stanford University, in a review of the efficacy of selected alternative treatments for unipolar depression, acupuncture was shown to be an effective alternative monotherapy for major depression.[8]

A survey conducted in Padua, Italy, found that acupuncture, among other alternative therapies, had a complementary role for the elderly with depressive symptoms.[9]

In a survey of complementary and alternative medicine (CAM) treatments, the University of Exeter found acupuncture for anxiety useful to cancer patients.[10]

AMINO ACIDS AND TRYPTOPHAN

Amino acids are building blocks of protein molecules and play a role in the production of mood-regulating brain neurotransmitters. The most important one is tryptophan (L-TP), a precursor to serotonin. But don't be fooled into thinking that just by eating a high protein diet you will get enough tryptophan, and therefore enough serotonin. In order for tryptophan to reach the brain and be converted into serotonin, it must first attach itself to a certain carrier molecule. Protein meals supply the body with several amino acids, not just tryptophan. And all of these amino acids are competing for a ride on the same carrier. Unfortunately, tryptophan is the least abundant of the amino acids and gets pushed aside by other amino acids, which bully their way onto the transport molecule. As a result, high-protein meals cause both tryptophan and serotonin levels to decline. On the other hand, complete carbohydrate meals, which don't contain tryptophan, are capable of producing a rapid and considerable increase in serotonin levels. Or meals with both protein and carbohydrates also raise serotonin. Turkey is high in tryptophan, just think of all the napping and dozing that goes on after a high-protein, high-carbohydrate, Thanksgiving dinner. Carbohydrates perform this transport function by stimulating the release of insulin. Insulin increases the ratio of available tryptophan, making the carrier molecule more accessible and causing increased tryptophan uptake.

The amino acid tryptophan is the precursor to serotonin and was used in the 1980s as a treatment for mild to moderate depression. It was in direct competition with Prozac, which was released in 1987. But, then in 1989 tryptophan was pulled from the market because it was thought to be the cause of Eosiniphilia myalgia syndrome, which in the United States caused thirty-seven deaths and left over 5,000 permanently disabled. It wasn't long before the real culprit was found, a new genetically-engineered binder added to a tryptophan formulation by a Japanese company. Over $2 billion has been paid in damages by the Japanese manufacturing company. However, tryptophan is still blamed as the cause of the Eosiniphilia myalgia outbreak and has been unavailable to the public ever since. Even though tryptophan is no longer available 5 hydroxytryptophan (5-HTP), derived from a natural plant source (griffonia simplicifolia), is found in health food stores and. Tryptophan is the direct precursor to 5-HTP which is immediately converted to serotonin. Doses of 50-100mg three times a day can boost brain serotonin levels enough to improve mood, calm anxiety, diminish compulsive behavior, reduce PMS, suppress appetite, decrease carbohydrate craving, improve sleep, and relieve headaches and symptoms of fibromyalgia. These are all the things that serotonin is supposed to do naturally, if we give it the right building blocks. The manufacturers of SSRIs don't want you to know this.

In 1978 Acta Psychiatric Scand published a study that claimed 5-HTP did not have an antidepressant effect, and that L-TP, without interacting pharmaca, did not appear to be a well-documented antidepressant.[11] However, this study has been superceded by more recent studies positive for L-TP.

A study in Vancouver found that rapid tryptophan depletion appears to reverse the antidepressant effect of bright light therapy in patients with seasonal affective disorder.[12]

A study in the United Arab Emirates found that multiple regression analysis showed a significant contribution for low tryptophan to increased Edinburgh postnatal depression (EPDS) on day 7 after delivery.[13]

After a number of studies challenged the findings that acute tryptophan depletion (TD) increases depressive symptoms in medicated, formerly depressed patients, a study in Boston found that the mood effect of TD in medicated, formerly depressed patients was confirmed. It suggested a threshold may exist for mood effects following TD, implying that recent negative findings may have been caused by insufficient depletion.[14]

Another study in the Netherlands demonstrated that repeated moderate TRP depletion leads to anxiogenic and depressive-like behavior in the rat and corroborates the notion of the involvement of serotonin in these behaviors.[15]

Alterations in brain tryptophan levels cause changes in brain serotonin synthesis, and this has been used to study the implication of altered serotonin levels in humans. A study in Canada showed that, overall, studies manipulating tryptophan levels support the idea that low serotonin can predispose subjects to mood and impulse control disorders, and higher levels of serotonin may help to promote more constructive social interactions by decreasing aggression and increasing dominance.[16]

Tyrosine is another amino acid that is the precursor to an important neurotransmitter, DOPA. It is also a precursor to adrenaline, thyroid hormones, and estrogen. Studies have shown that it lowers blood pressure, suppresses appetite and increases sex drive. But, because it is a precursor to adrenaline it could make a manic episode worse so it should not be used for the treatment of manic depression. The average dose is 500mg three times a day. Some feel that more should not be taken without the advice of a health care practitioner. Too much tyrosine may trigger migraine headaches.

Phenylalanine is the amino acid precursor to tyrosine and has been used to treat depression. It should not be used, however, by people who have phenylketonuria (PKU), a genetic disorder that makes it impossible for the body to break down phenylalanine. PKU is usually diagnosed at birth and since a mother does not know if her child could have PKU phenylalanine supplements should be avoided in pregnancy. The dosage for phenylalanine is 500 mg three times a day.

Phosphatidylserine is an amino acid which works through the hypothalamus to regulate the amount of cortisone produced by the adrenals. Stressful events cause an increase in cortisone in the blood stream which can keep people on edge and sleepless and lead to depression. Phosphatidylserine helps support and restores nerve cells, and numerous studies show that it slows or reverses cognitive losses attributed to aging.

An article in the Alternative Medical Review presents a survey of nutrients and botanicals in the integrative management of cognitive dysfunction and found that phosphatidylserine improved mood in middle-aged and elderly subjects with dementia or age-related cognitive decline.[17]

AROMATHERAPY

Aromatherapy, as one of our studies shows, is a burgeoning new healing modality used by nurses. Concentrated oils from plants are rubbed into the skin for a variety of complaints. These oils contain powerful antioxidants that are absorbed through the skin into the blood stream and can have medicinal effects on the body. The following studies show that certain oils can have profound effects on anxiety and mood.

The University of Southampton determined that Lavender oil administered in an aroma stream showed modest efficacy in the treatment of agitated behavior in patients with severe dementia.[18]

In a study at a hospital in Reading, England, patients who received aromatherapy reported significantly greater improvement in their mood and perceived levels of anxiety.[19]

A study in England demonstrated that aromatherapy can be effective in reducing maternal anxiety, fear and/or pain during labour.[20]

A survey in Seattle, Washington, found that aromatherapy is the fastest growing of all complementary therapies among nurses in the United States.[21]

A study in California found that antioxidants such as eugenol and maltol play an important role in the pharmaceutical activities of natural plant extracts used for aromatherapy.[22]

AYURVEDA

Individual herbs and herbal formulas used in Ayurveda, the classical system of Indian medicine, have proven successful in the treatment of depression. For example, a study in Varanasi, India, showed that bioactive glycowithanolides (WSG), isolated from the roots of Withania somnifera, induced an anxiolytic effect, comparable to that produced by lorazepam, in rats. WSG also exhibited an antidepressant effect, comparable with that induced by imipramine, in the forced swim-induced "behavioral despair" and "learned helplessness" tests in the rats.[23]

Another study in Varanasi, India, showed that an Ayurveda herbal formulation Siotone (ST) reversed the chronic stress-induced increase in rat brain tribulin activity, demonstrating attributes similar to the modern concept of adaptogenic agents which are known to afford protection of the human physiological system against diverse stressors.[24]

Significant antianxiety effects were induced in rats by low doses of the leaf extract of Azadirachta indica that were comparable to those induced by diazepam.[25]

BACH FLOWER REMEDIES

In a survey conducted in the United Kingdom of CAM-providers representing twelve therapies, it was deemed that stress/anxiety was the most common condition alleviated.[26]

BALNEOTHERAPY

Balneotherpay is a general term for water-based treatments using natural spring, mineral or seawater to encourage relaxation, improve the circulation, stimulate the immune system, and revitalize and detoxify the body.

Even simple actions as foot-bathing for ten minutes in hot

water, with or without the addition of essential oil of lavender, can produce beneficial effects. For example, researchers in Japan found the foot-bath produced a significant increase in blood flow. And in the case of the foot-bath with the addition of essential oil of lavender, there were delayed changes to the balance of autonomic activity in the direction associated with relaxation.[27]

Italians found a statistically significant reduction in anxiety and somatisation parameters with arsenic-iron bath treatment for subjects suffering from endogenous reactive anxiety syndromes with somatisation.[28]

A study in Turkey showed that balneotherapy is effective in treating the pain and anxiety of fibromyalgia patients.[29]

In Spain, researchers found that sadness as a feeling of disproportional affective reaction with mental consequences can find relief in Spa cures, or balneotherapy.[30]

A study in Israel found that patients with fibromyalgia were relieved during a ten-day stay at a Dead Sea spa.[31]

BIBLIOTHERAPY

Bibliotherapy in the form of self-help books, self-help internet sites, or printed material from health-care professionals goes a long way to helping people deal with their feelings of anxiety, stress, and depression.

At the University of Pennsylvania the importance of minimal therapist contact by patients when coupled with manual-based bibliotherapy interventions (such as self-help books, electronic database searches, correspondence with authors and limited handsearching) led to significant reductions on measures of frequency of panic attacks, panic cognitions, anticipatory anxiety, and depression.[32]

Researchers in Australia found that Web sites are a practical and promising means of delivering cognitive behavioral interventions for preventing depression and anxiety to the general public.[33]

Less contact with therapists proves beneficial if patients are supported in learning skills to manage their symptoms (assisted bibliotherapy) from moderate anxiety disorders.[34]

Behavior problems in children are quite common and many approaches such as medication are limited due to factors such as time and expense. In the U.K. it was found that media-based interventions (bibliotherapy) had both clinical and economic advantages as regards the treatment of children with behavioral problems.[35]

Other studies show a wide range of alternatives to counter the negative side effects of conventional medication treatments for depression. For example, calcium is the most abundant mineral in the body. It has profound effects on the nervous system and mood.

CALCIUM

In Rhode Island a study reported that calcium was effective in reducing emotional, behavioral, and physical premenstrual symptoms.[36]

In New York City, oral calcium supplementation reversed the reduced vitamin B12 absorption that metformin induced in patients with depression.[37]

CHOLESTEROL

Despite the fact that most people are worried about having cholesterol levels that are too high, yet another study has found that low cholesterol is actually associated with adverse behavioral effects such as aggression and depression.[38]

COGNITIVE-BEHAVIORAL THERAPY

Cognitive-behavioral therapy (CBT) is the most thoroughly studied nonpharmacologic approach to the treatment of social anxiety disorder, and its efficacy has been demonstrated in a large number of investigations.[39]

At Stanford University, CBT was shown to result in statistically significant reductions of performance anxiety in musicians whereas buspirone was not an effective treatment.[40]

Another study in California of generalized anxiety disorder (GAD) recommended that clinicians should consider the potential benefits of psychotherapy as an adjunct to medication.[41]

Researchers in Albany found that patients showed significant improvement in quality of life scores after completion of cognitive-behavioral group therapy for social phobia.[42]

In Rhode Island , a study showed the efficacy of cognitive therapy in the treatment of premenstrual syndrome.[43]

However, CBT, along with other verbal psychosocial treatments for anxiety disorders, has declined in use in the nineties.[44]

A study reported in Psychopathology recommended that color therapy could be used to follow changes in the state of depressive patients and to predict their response to anti-depressant pharmacotherapy.[15]

In the Netherlands a study indicated that the colors of antidepressant drugs affected the perceived action of the drug and seemed to influence the effectiveness of the drug.[46]

In Seattle a computer program (Computer Assisted Relaxation Learning) for conducting exposure therapy for the treatment of dental injection fear, which trained subjects to use physical and cognitive relaxation techniques, was found to reduce their general fear of dental injections.[47]

DHEA

Standard replacement for adrenal insufficiency consists of gluco-corticoids and mineralocorticoids while dehydroepiandrosterone (DHEA) deficiency is routinely ignored. However, in Germany, a study demonstrated that DHEA treatment significantly improved overall wellbeing as well as scores for depression, anxiety, and their physical correlates in women with adrenal insufficiency.[48]

A survey conducted in U.L.B. found that recent studies show DHEA supplementation has proven beneficial in typical deficient states like adrenal insufficiency or major depressive illnesses.[49]

A study reported in the American Journal of Psychiatry found that elevated cortisol-DHEA ratios may be a state marker of depressive illness and may contribute to the associated deficits in learning and memory. It recommended that administration of DHEA may reduce neurocognitive deficits in major depression.[50]

At the University of Cambridge a study found that increased negative mood and feelings and DHEA hypersecretion at entry were associated with subsequent first-episode major depression in adolescents.[51]

In Japan the data in a study suggested a possibility that endoge-nous DHEA sulphate and dietary soy may modulate psychologic well-being of peri- and postmenopausal women.[52]

Another study at the University of Cambridge demonstrated that lower DHEA levels are an additional state of abnormality in adult depression.[53]

At the University of Pittsburgh a study suggested that the decrease in DHEA and DHEA-S remitters is related to remission of depression rather than to a direct drug effect on steroids.[54]

Because of the recent large quantities of DHEA sold in health food stores, a team at the University of Cambridge undertook a thorough investigation of well-conducted studies of DHEA supplementation for cognition and well-being, and they found the data offered support for the claimed improvement in a sense of well-being following DHEA treatment.[55]

DIET

The body is built from what we eat, drink, and breathe. If we choose the cleanest and most healthy food and drink we have a better chance of building a healthy body. If we choose synthetic, processed foods we increase our chances of ill health because those foods are mostly devoid of nutrients. Vitamins and minerals from healthy food sources provide the necessary co-factors required by all the enzymes in the body. Enzymes run metabolic processes including essential neurotransmitter production and function in the brain. Without the proper building blocks and nutrients these neurotransmitters malfunction resulting in mood and behavior problems.

In Seattle a study demonstrated that psychological distress is associated with unhealthful dietary practices.[56]

In the U.K. researchers found that the presence of depression was the most powerful predictor of levels of well-being, but the finding of a high body mass index is likely to indicate adequate well-being of older people.[57]

In Germany a study showed that dietary treatment cannot be neglected as a possible access to treating hyperactive/disruptive children and merits further investigation. [58]

A series of studies in Norway suggested a correlation between somatic and neuropsychiatric symptoms and emotional disturbances, and they noted that patients identifying themselves as sensitive to food and chemicals had higher scores for depression, anxiety, shyness, and defensiveness.[59]

A survey in the U.K. revealed that certain dietary risk factors for physical ill health are also risk factors for depression and cognitive impairment. For example, cognitive impairment is associated with atherosclerosis, type 2 diabetes and hypertension, and findings from a broad range of studies showed significant relationships between cognitive function and intakes of various nutrients, including long-chain polyunsaturated fatty acids, antioxidant vitamins, and folate and vitamin B12.[60]

A recent review summarizing the most important research, particularly that from 1985 to 1995, on the relationship between diet and behavior concluded that diet definitely affects some children. Symptoms which changed included those seen in attention deficit disorder (ADD) and attention deficit hyperactivity disorder (ADHD), sleep problems, physical symptoms, with later research emphasizing particularly changes in mood.[61]

DRUMMING

Drumming is a recent therapeutic technique that comes to us from aboriginal cultures. A study conducted in Pennsylvania found that group drumming music therapy is a complex composite intervention with the potential to modulate specific neuroendocrine and neuroimmune parameters in a direction opposite to that expected with the classic stress response.[62]

ESSENTIAL FATTY ACIDS

Essential Fatty Acids (EFAs) are also called Vitamin F, designating the nutritional aspects of fats and oils. Essential means that we all need certain amounts of these fats for optimum health. With regard to mental health EFAs maintain and enhance normal brain development and functioning. EFAs are also building blocks for hormone-like substances called prostaglandins that regulate immune system functions and play a central role in stress reduction.

There are two main essential fatty acids: Omega-3 fatty acids and Omega-6 fatty acids. Omega-3 fatty acids are also called alpha linoleic acids found in flax and hemp oils. Omega-6 fatty acids are called linoleic acid found in flax, hemp, borage, and evening primrose oils. Other non-essential but healthy oils are: Eicosapentaenoic acid (RPA) found in fish oil; Docosahexaenoic acid (DHA) found in fish oil; and gamma linolenic acid (GLA) found in borage, hemp, and evening primrose oil.

Evening primrose oil extracted from the primrose plant is high in an omega-6 essential fatty acid called gamma linoleic acid.

An article in the Journal of Reproductive Medicine reports that three studies all demonstrated that evening primrose oil is a highly effective treatment for the depression and irritability associated with premenstrual syndrome.[63]

A study in Boston found that Omega3 fatty acids were well tolerated and improved the short-term course of illness in patients with bipolar disorder.[64]

An article in Biological Psychiatry reports that a study showed that three behaviorally different mental disorders were ameliorated with supplements of a newly discovered trace omega-3 essential fatty acid (w3-EFA).[65]

A team in Japan previously found that DHA intake prevented aggression enhancement at times of mental stress. In this study they investigated changes in aggression under nonstressful conditions and found that aggression levels remained stable in the DHA group.[66]

EXERCISE

From the runner's high, which stimulates a rush of adrenaline, to the calming effects of a walk through the woods, exercise has the power to lift one's spirits.

A survey in Norway found beneficial psychological effects of exercise are best documented for mild to moderate forms of unipolar depression, and in panic and generalized anxiety disorders. It is suggested a simple and inexpensive approach like exercise is helpful and might be important for public health.[67]

In an Australian survey of complementary and self-help treatments for depression, exercise was cited as one of several having the best evidence of effectiveness.[68]

In California a study found that a twelve-month exercise program for women who were caring for relatives with dementia increased knowledge of the benefits of exercise, increased motivational readiness for exercise, and alleviated perceived stress, burden, and depression. The study demonstrated the feasibility and success of delivering home-based health promotion counseling for improving physical activity levels in a highly stressed and burdened population.[69]

FLAVONOIDS

Bioflavonoids, or flavonoids, are plant pigments found in all plants.

The data collected in this paper from Argentina makes clear that some natural flavonoids are CNS-active molecules and that the chemical modification of the flavone nucleus dramatically increases their anxiolytic potency – in one case creating a drug 30 times more potent than diazepam.[70]

Another study in Argentina found that Tilia species, traditional medicinal plants widely used in Latin America as sedatives and tranquilizers, extracted in a complex fraction containing as yet unidentified constituents probably of a flavonoid nature, when administered in mice, had a clear anxiolytic effect but no effect on total and ambulatory locomotor activity.[71]

In Germany a study found that the antidepressant effect of apocynum leaves on male rats in a forced swimming test indicated antidepressant activity comparable to the tricyclic antidepressant imipramine. It further speculated that this effect might be related to hyperoside and isoquercitrin which are major flavonoids in the extract.[72]

FOLIC ACID

Folic acid is a member of the Vitamin B family and is well known for its ability to prevent birth defects in infants when taken during pregnancy. An article in The Townsend Letter for Doctors and Patients reported on a study whose results indicated that supplementation with folic acid may increase the efficacy and reduce the side effects of fluoxetine in women with depression. Patients with depression have consistently been found to have low plasma and RBC folate levels, and low plasma folate has been associated with a poor response to antidepressant medications.[73]

GUIDED IMAGERY

Guided Imagery refers to a number of techniques including simple visualization or a direct suggestion. The mental image formed in a guided imagery session may be seen, heard, tasted, smelled, touched, or felt. Therapeutic guided imagery allows patients to experience a relaxed state of mind and then focus on images associated with their problems. A dialogue is then created with their problem out of which often come answers and understanding. Or, simple visualization can take one on a relaxing journey to a safe place in nature and help diminish stress.

The Holistic Nursing Practitioner reported on a study that found that subjects who listened to a guided imagery/relaxation tape before their magnetic resonance imaging (MRI) scan had lower levels of anxiety and moved less during the MRI scan.[74]

A study in Louisiana revealed that surgical patients listening to Relaxation with Guided Imagery (RGI) audiotapes demonstrated significantly less state anxiety, lower cortisol levels one day following surgery, and less surgical wound erythema.[75]

In Kansas a study found that guided imagery lowered the anxiety levels of nursing students learning to perform their first injections and recommended introduction of this teaching strategy early in the curriculum.[76]

Researchers in Philadelphia found that guided imagery was well-received by bereaved spouses with promising psychoimmunological trends that merited more rigorous investigation.[77]

A study in Miami showed that guided imagery and music (GIM), when used on healthy adults, resulted in significant decreases between pre- and postsession depression, fatigue, and total mood disturbance, and had significant decreases in cortisol level by follow-up. It suggested such changes in hormonal regulation may have health implications for chronically stressed people.[78]

An article in the Journal of Holistic Nursing reports how guided imagery protocol applied to the first 4 weeks of the postpartum period resulted in less anxiety and depression and greater self-esteem in primiparas.[79]

The Annual Review of Nursing published a review of 46 studies of the use of guided imagery in the management of stress, anxiety, and depression published between 1966 and 1998 which pointed to preliminary evidence of its effectiveness.[80]

A study at the Group/Walther Cancer Institute explored the effectiveness of guided imagery in alleviating mood disturbance and improving quality of life in cancer patients. The results indicated it significantly improved mood and quality of life in these cancer patients.[81]

A study published in the Journal of Gerontology Nursing indicated that discharge teaching using guided imagery has the potential to decrease depression in older adults after discharge from the hospital.[82]

HERBS

Herbal medicine has a much larger role in Europe in the treatment of mood disorders than in the United States. The most important mood-balancing herb is St. John's Wort. It has antidepressant, anti-anxiety, and sedative properties as well as being a strong anti-inflammatory. Research indicates that its antidepressant effects are due to its serotonin reuptake inhibition properties, which keep serotonin levels elevated. This is the same mechanism by which Prozac works, but without the side effects.

Many other herbs are effective in treating depression and anxiety. In Germany one study showed that a unique extract of black cohosh is associated with improvement in menopause symptoms, including mood changes, without evidence of estrogen-like effects.[83]

A study in India reports that ginkgolic acid conjugates (GAC) isolated from the leaves of Indian Ginkgo biloba showed consistent and significant anxiolytic activity in rats.[84]

A team in Ottawa, Canada, found that Gotu Kola attenuated

the peak acoustic startle response (ASR) in healthy human subjects after earlier studies showed that Gotu Kola decreased locomotor activity and attenuated ASR in rats.[85]

Researchers in Germany did a study that confirmed the anxiolytic efficacy and good tolerance of kava-kava special extract WS1490 and also showed that a further symptom reduction is possible after a change-over from benzodiazepine treatment.[86]

A study at the Duke University Medical Center suggested that kava-kava might exert a favourable effect on reflex vagal control of heart rate in generalized anxiety disorder patients.[87]

A study in London demonstrated that kava-kava relieved total stress severity as well as stress-induced insomnia.[88]

Also in the U.K. an extensive review of published and unpublished studies of Kava-kava extract implied it is superior to placebo and relatively safe as a symptomatic treatment for anxiety.[89]

In Germany researchers found that Kava pyrones exhibit a profile of cellular actions that shows a large overlap with several mood stabilizers, especially lamotrigine.[90]

A study in Basel found that there were no residual sedative effects (hangover) on the morning after ingestion of valerian extracts as compared to the morning after ingestion of benzodiazepines where there was impairment of vigilance.[91]

A study in Japan of the psychotropic effects of Japanese valerian root extract found that it acts on the central nervous system and may be an antidepressant.[92].

A study in the United Kingdom found that valerian may be beneficial to health by reducing physiological reactivity during stressful situations.[93]

HOMEOPATHY

Homeopathy is a medical practice that uses extremely dilute

plant or mineral substances, which have no side effects. Some individual homeopathic medicines can be prescribed for acute conditions, such as aconite, which is specific for fear and terror. However, for symptoms of depression it is often more beneficial for the individual to see a homeopath for a detailed history and prescription of the specific remedy for his or her case.

A study in France showed that aconite proved to be effective for children's postoperative agitation with 95% good results.[94]

HYPNOSIS

An article in the American Journal of Clinical Hypnosis summarized aspects of effective psychotherapy for major depression and described how hypnosis is helpful in reducing common symptoms of major depression such as agitation and rumination and thereby may decrease a client's sense of helplessness and hopelessness. It stated that hypnosis is also effective in facilitating the learning of new skills, a core component of all empirically supported treatments for major depression.[95]

A study in India found that hypnosis and a later follow-up period of self-hypnosis removed chronic repeated episodes of stress-related hemoptysis in a 24-year-old patient.[96]

A study in London demonstrated the sizeable influences on cell-mediated immunity achieved by a relatively brief, low cost psychological intervention (self-hypnosis) in the face of a compelling, but routine, stress in young, healthy adults that has implications for illness prevention and for patients with compromised immunity.[97]

INOSITOL

Inositol is a member of the Vitamin B family.

A study in Israel compared inositol, a natural isomer of glucose, with an established drug, fluvoxamine, in the treatment of panic disorder. Inosital reduced the greater number of panic attacks per week and proved attractive to patients because it is a natural compound with few known side effects.[98]

A second study in Israel found that inositol was effective as sole therapy for depression, and proved as effective as imipramine in treating panic disorder.[99]

LAUGHTER

A team in Japan found that natural killer cell activity (NKCA) elevation and NKCA before and after comic film seem to be related with the experiential aspects of laughter rather than with the expressive aspects.[100]

LIGHT THERAPY

A study at Yale University found that morning light therapy has an antidepressant effect during pregnancy.[101]

In Vancouver researchers found that an active bright white light condition significantly reduced depression and pre-menstrual tension during the symptomatic luteal phase in women with late luteal phase dysphoric disorder (LLPDD).[102]

Seasonal affective disorder (SAD) is the name given to people who get depressed when they don't get enough natural sunlight.

A study in Sweden found that light therapy with concomitant and continued SSRI (citalopram) treatment is a useful strategy to achieve beneficial long-term effects in patients with seasonal affective disorder (SAD).[103]

A study in Finland indicated that bright light administered twice a week, alone or combined with physical exercise, seemed to be a useful intervention for relieving seasonal mood slumps.[104]

A study in The Netherlands demonstrated that bright light therapy had a positive effect on motor restless behaviour in patients with dementia.[105]

MAGNETIC STIMULATION

Our heart and brain emit the most electromagnetism in the body. The heart's energy is measured by the electrocardiogram, and the brain's energy is measured by the electroencephalogram. Knowing the electromagnetic potential of the brain, many researchers have tried to manufacture devices to try to "balance" the brain's electromagnetic output. The following series of studies show the benefits of such intervention:

A study in Chicago compared repetitive transcranial magnetic stimulation (rTMS), a noninvasive technique to modulate cortical excitability, to electroconvulsive therapy (ECT) in severely ill, depressed patients and found comparable therapeutic effects.[106]

An article in the American Journal of Psychiatry reviews studies of "slow" rTMS and finds slow rTMS offers a new method for probing and possibly treating brain hyperexcitability syndromes.[107]

In the U.K. another review of studies of the effectiveness of rTMS indicated its demonstrable beneficial effects in the treatment of depression.[108]

A study in Iowa found that rTMS improved significantly the cognitive flexibility and conceptual tracking of middle-aged and elderly patients with refractory depression.[109]

In Germany a report was published that described the treatment of a patient with major depression who had been hospitalized for 60 months during a period of 7 years with no improvement, even from electroconvulsive therapy, but once treated with rTMS was discharged after just 4 weeks of daily treatment.[110]

MEDITATION

Prayer, self-reflection, chanting, and meditation all have a soothing and calming effect on the psyche.

A study in Philadelphia concluded that a group mindfulness meditation training program can enhance functional status and well-being and reduce physical symptoms and psychological distress in a heterogeneous patient population and that the intervention may have long-term beneficial effects.[111]

A study in Canada found that a mindfulness meditation-based stress reduction program was effective in decreasing mood disturbance and stress symptoms in both male and female patients with a wide variety of cancer diagnoses, stages of illness, and ages.[112]

Another study in Arizona investigated the short-term effects of an 8-week meditation-based stress reduction intervention on pre-medical and medical students and found that participation in the intervention could reduce self-reported state and trait anxiety, reduce reports of overall psychological distress including depression, increase scores on overall empathy levels, and increase scores on a measure of spiritual experiences at termination of intervention.[113]

MELATONIN

Melatonin is a hormone produced by the pineal gland and is responsible for our sleeping/waking cycle. It is elevated at night before bedtime and lowest in the morning. It has become a common sleep aid. By helping people get a good night's rest it can lesson symptoms of anxiety and depression.

A pilot study in Argentina suggested that melatonin can be an alternative and safe treatment for patients with fibromyalgia. Adverse events were mild and transient.[114]

Benzodiazepines are the most frequently used drug for the treatment of insomnia. However, prolonged use of benzodiazepine therapy is not recommended. A study in Israel found that controlled-release melatonin effectively facilitated discontinuation of benzodiazepine therapy while maintaining good sleep quality.[115]

MIND-BODY MEDICINE

The field of psychoneuroimmunology is successfully bridging the mind-body split in light of recent research that finds brain neurotransmitters and their effects in the gut and throughout the whole lymphatic system. This means our gut and, in effect, our whole body, can experience moods, which may be expressed as physical symptoms but are a direct effect of a shift in our emotions.

A review published in Gerontology found that there was significant impact of affective disorders on immune functions in the elderly subjects. Due to the high frequency in the aged of autoimmune, infectious, and neoplastic diseases it recommended a focus on the psychoneuroimmune interactions in old age.[116]

A study in Ohio found that production of protoinflammatory cytokines that influence conditions associated with aging can be directly stimulated by negative emotions and stressful experiences. Additionally, negative emotions also contributed to prolonged infection and delayed wound healing, processes that fuel sustained proinflammatory cytokine production.[117]

A review conducted in Australia found that a number of studies have demonstrated that stress increases the risk of viral infection, and stress and depression can depress immunity whereas stress reduction can enhance immunity.[118]

A study in South Africa found that acute phase proteins were significantly raised in a group of patients with depressive disorder and suggested there was an interaction between psychological state and immune systems operative in host defenses.[119]

An article in Semin Clin Neuropsychiatry reviewed evidence that showed a bi-directional relationship between the brain and the immune system. These findings implicated a role for the immune system in the cause of behavioral disorders in a wide range of medical illnesses. And a paradigm was proposed in which abnormal functioning of either the hypothalamic-pituitary-adrenal (HPA) axis or the inflammatory response system disrupts feedback regulation of both neuroendocrine and immune systems contributing to the development of neuropsychiatric and immunologic disorders.[120]

A study in Japan investigated the relationship between the psychological and immunological state in patients with atopic dermatitis and found that patients with atopic dermatitis were significantly more depressive and scored higher for state anxiety. The study concluded that the psychological state is related to the immunological state.[121]

A second study in Japan reports that recent psychoneuroimmunological research demonstrates that depression or other types of emotional stress damages the immune system, which can induce some physical diseases, especially for the elderly, who have weakened cell-mediated immune function and are more susceptible to influence by the damaged immune function caused by such psychiatric dysfunction.[122]

In San Francisco a review of clinical trials of mind-body medicine (MBM) techniques found that certain MBM therapies are effective in improving quality of life, anxiety, and pain intensity for a variety of conditions.[123]

MUSIC THERAPY

It was after both world wars that music therapy gained prominence as local musicians were hired by hospitals to play music for shell-shocked soldiers. The response to music by anxious and depressed patients has been well documented over the decades.

An article in Intensive Crit Care Nurs discusses a study in which patients waiting for their cardiac catheterization benefited from music therapy. Anxiety and the heightened physiological values elicited by the stress response were reduced. Results also suggested that women waiting for cardiac catheterization experience a higher level of anxiety than males.[124]

A study in Italy found that proctological patients who listened to a guided imagery tape with music and relaxing text before, during, and after surgery experienced reduced pain following anorectal surgery and improved quality of sleep.[125]

In Norway an overview of central areas of application of music in clinical medicine found music has been used successfully to treat anxiety and depression and improve function in schizophrenia and autism. The supportive role of music has a natural field of application in palliative medicine and terminal care.[126]

PHOTOTHERAPY

A study in France found that phototherapy has been a successful alternative treatment to medication, in addition to antidepressive medication, and as primary treatment of seasonal depression.[127]

PSYCHODRAMA

Psychodrama is a form of therapy where patients act out scenarios of life events that give them insight into their problems.

A study in Massachusetts found that psychodrama groups with traumatized middle-school girls revealed significant decreases in group participants' self-reported difficulties in withdrawn behavior and anxiety/depression.[128]

A review of three trials in the United Kingdom found that psychological intervention in the form of psychodynamic psychotherapy may be useful in the treatment of non-ulcer dyspepsia.[129]

REIKI

Reiki is a form of bodywork that is actually an ancient natural healing art patterned after the healings performed by Jesus. Reiki uses a laying on of hands system of touch healing. It promotes healing on all levels: physical, mental, emotional, and spiritual.

An article in the Journal of Indian Med Assoc. has outlined the contemporary application of Reiki principles to the physical response to stress and stress related illnesses.[130]

RELIGION

Dr. Larry Dossey has written a book, The Power of Prayer, citing volumes of research that prove the power of prayer to heal both physical and emotional imbalance.

A review of studies published in the Int J Psychiatry Med found that if religious beliefs and practices improve coping, reduce stress, prevent or facilitate the resolution of depression, improve social support, promote healthy behaviors, and prevent alcohol and drug abuse, then a plausible mechanism exists by which physical health may be affected.[131]

REMINISCENCE THERAPY

A study in North Carolina demonstrated that reminiscence therapy is an effective means of reducing depression among institutionalized, rural-dwelling elders, especially older women, who resist treatment from mental health services for a variety of different reasons.[132]

THERAPEUTIC TOUCH

Therapeutic touch is defined as the sharing of life force energies between two or more people with the intent of causing a healing transformation physically and spiritually. It involves light touching to direct healing energy.

A study in Alabama found that therapeutic touch (TT), an intervention in which human energies are therapeutically manipulated, versus sham TT could produce greater pain relief as an adjunct to narcotic analgesia, a greater reduction in anxiety, and alterations in plasma T-lymphocyte concentrations among burn patients.[133]

A study in Quebec, Canada, showed that TT treatments increased the sensation of well-being and reduced depression and anxiety in persons with terminal cancer.[134]

A study in New York State found that five postpartum women who participated in therapeutic touch during home visits for 2 months experienced many positive emotions.[135]

An article in J Holist Nurs discussed the beneficial effects of TT on seven hospitalized, adolescent psychiatric patients who received a total of 31 TT treatments over two 2-week periods.[136]

THERMAL THERAPY

A study in Italy showed that data on females and males with no psychiatric history, attending thermal facilities while testing for their psychoneurotic profiles, supported the hypothesis that a particular form of neurosis, in particular gastrointestinal referred somatic disease, may play a significant role in motivating request of thermal therapies.[137]

VITAMINS

A study in California of the effect of thiamin (vitamin B1) supplementaton proved positive for nonspecific conditions such as anorexia, weight loss, fatigue, sleep disorders, and depression in an elderly Irish population with marginal thiamin deficiency.[138]

In New York State 24 chronic schizophrenic patients were treated successfully with the addition of acetazolamide and thiamine to their unchanged existing therapies.[139]

A study in Germany examined whether patients with Alzheimer's disease (AD) with subnormal vitamin B12 levels show more frequent behavioral and psychological symptoms of dementia than AD patients with normal vitamin B12 levels. The results show vitamin B12 could play a role in the pathogenesis of behavioral changes in AD.[140]

REFERENCES

CHAPTER TWO

1. Vedantam S. Washington Post, January 9, 2002; Page A01
2. Vedantam S. Washington Post, May 21, 2002; Page A01
3. Ann Landers website
4. Screening for Mental Health, Inc. website
5. Screening for Mental Health, Inc. website
6. Nintendo Neurology, Scientific American, August 2000.

CHAPTER THREE

1. *The Hoax of Learning and Behavior Disorders,* Citizens Commission on Human Rights (pamphlet), Los Angeles, 2001.
2. Zito, Julie Magno, "Trends in the Prescribing of Psychotropic Medications to Preschoolers," *Journal of the American Medical Association*, Feb. 23, 2000, Vol. 283, No. 8, pp. 1025–30.
3. West, Jean, "Children's drug is more potent than cocaine," *The Observer*, London, Sept. 9, 2001.
4. Graham, J.E., et al., "A double-blind, randomized, placebo-controlled trial of fluoxetine in children and adolescents with depression." *Arch. Gen. Psychiatry*, 1997; 54:1031–37.
5. Breggin, Peter R., "Today's Kids Suffer Legal Drug Abuse," *Newsday*, Sept. 23, 1999, p. A53.
6. Gary Null interview with Dr. Fred Baughman, Feb. 12, 2001.
7. DeGrandpre, Richard, *Ritalin Nation*, W.W. Norton & Co., New York, 1999, p. 160.
8. Elkind, David, *The Hurried Child*, Addison-Wesley, New York, 1981.
9. Suriano, Robyn, "As kids get put on pills, critics fret," *Orlando Sentinel*, Nov. 26, 2001.
10. Gary Null interview with Dr. David Stein, Feb. 13, 2001.

References

11. *Ibid.*
12. Suriano, *op. cit.*
13. Harris, Gardiner, "Use of Mood-Altering Drugs to Control Toddlers' Behavior Jumped in the '90s," *Wall Street Journal*, Fed. 23, 2000.
14. Zito, Julie Magno, "Trends in the Prescribing of Psychotropic Medications to Preschoolers," *Journal of the American Medical Association*, Feb. 23, 2000, Vol. 283, No. 8, pp. 1025–30.
15. Robinson, Holly, "Generation Rx," *Parents*, Nov. 2001, p. 82.
16. Kaiser, David, "Commentary: Against Biologic Psychiatry," *Psychiatric Times*, CME Inc., *webmaster@mhsource.com*.
17. O'Meara, Kelly Patricia, "Writing May Be on Wall for Ritalin," *Insight*, Oct. 16, 2000, *omeara@insightmag.com*.
18. Zernike, Kate, and Melody Peterson, "Schools' Backing of Behavior Drugs Comes Under Fire," *The New York Times*, Aug. 19, 2001.
19. Breggin, Peter R., *Talking Back to Ritalin: What Doctors Aren't Telling You About Stimulants for Children*, Common Courage Press, Monroe, ME, 1998, p. 5.
20. Lipkin, P.H., et al., "Tics and dyskinesias associated with stimulant treatment in attention-deficit hyperactivity disorder," *Arch. Pediatr. Adolesc. Med.*, Aug. 1994, 148(8):859–61.
21. Gerlach, J., et al., "Methylphenidate, apomorphine, THIP, and diazepam in monkeys . . . dopamine-GABA behavior related to psychoses and tardive dyskinesia," *Psychopharmacology (Berl.)*, 1984, 82(1–2): 131–4.
22. Young, J.G., "Methylphenidate-induced hallucinosis: case histories and possible mechanisms of action," *J. Dev. Behav. Pediatr.*, June 1981, 2(2):35–8.
23. Weiner, W.J., et al., "Methylphenidate-induced chorea: case report and pharmacological implications," *Neurology*, Oct. 1978, 28(10): 1041–4.
24. Silver, Larry B., *Dr. Larry Silver's Advice to Parents on Attention-Deficit Hyperactivity Disorder*, American Psychiatric Press, Washington, D.C., 1993, p. 189.
25. Taylor, John F., *Helping Your Hyperactive/Attention Deficit Child*, Prima Publishing, Rocklin, CA, 1994, p. 87.
26. Sears, William, and Lynda Thompson, *The A.D.D. Book: New Understandings, New Approaches to Parenting Your Child*, Little, Brown and Co., New York, 1998, p. 235.
27. Taylor, John F., *Helping Your Hyperactive/Attention Deficit Child*, Prima Publishing, Rocklin, CA, 1994, p. 91.

References

28. Swanson, J.S., et al., "Stimulant medication and the treatment of children with attention deficit disorder: A Review of Reviews," *Exceptional Children*, 1993, Vol. 60, pp. 154–61.
29. Gary Null interview with Janet Hall, Feb.13, 2001.
30. *Ibid.*
31. Associated Press, "Ritalin Maker Sued Over Girl's Death," *The Record* (New Jersey), Jan. 9, 2000, p. A-3.
32. Gary Null interview with Janet Hall, Feb.13, 2001.
33. Gary Null interview with Dr. Dragovic, Feb.13, 2001.
34. *Ibid.*
35. Wang, G.J., et al., "Methylphenidate decreases regional cerebral blood flow in normal human subjects," *Life Sci.*, 1994, 54(9): PL143–6.
36. Suplee, Curt, "Brain not finished developing by age 6, scientists now say," *The Philadelphia Inquirer*, Mar. 9, 2000.
37. Henderson, T.A., and Fischer, V.W., "Effects of methylphenidate (Ritalin) on mammalian myocardial ultrastructure," *American Journal of Cardiovascular Pathology*, 1995, 5(1): 68–78.
38. Gary Null interview with Dr. Fred Baughman, Feb. 12, 2001.
39. DeGrandpre, *op. cit.*
40. *Ibid.*, p. 19.
41. Zernike, Kate, and Melody Peterson, "Schools' Backing of Behavior Drugs Comes Under Fire," *The New York Times*, Aug. 19, 2001.
42. Ziegler, Nicole, "Recreational Ritalin," The Associated Press, abcNEWS.com, May 5, 2000.
43. Clerman, G., ed., *Contemporary Directions in Psychopathology*, 1986.
44. Couchon, Dennis, "Patients often aren't informed of full danger," *USA Today*, Dec. 6, 1995.
45. Boodman, Sandra G., "Shock Therapy . . . It's Back," *The Washington Post*, Sept. 24, 1996, p. Z14.
46. Boodman, *op. cit.*
47. *Electroshock as Head Injury: Report for the National Head Injury Foundation*, Sept. 1991.
48. Samant, Sydney, *Clinical Psychiatry News*, Mar. 1983.
49. Freeman, C., and Kendell, R., "Patients' experience of and attitudes to electroconvulsive therapy," *Annals of the New York Academy of Sciences*, 462 (1986), 341–52.
50. Gerring, Joan P., and Shields, Helen M., "The identification and manage-

ment of patients with a high risk for cardiac arrhythmias during modified ECT," *J. Clin. Psychiatry*, 43–4.

51. Appendix to Breeding, John, "Electroshock." Based on an article in the *J. of Humanistic Psychology*, Winter 2000, Vol. 40, No. 1, pp. 65–69, citing Ali, P.B., and Tidmarsh,, M.D., Cardiac Rupture During Electroconvulsive Therapy Anesthesia 1997; 52: 884–895.

52. Boodman, *op. cit.*

53. Edelson, E., "ECT elicits controversy—and results," *Houston Chronicle*, Dec. 28, 1988, p.3, as reported in "Electroshock: Death, Brain Damage, Memory Loss, and Brainwashing," *op. cit.*, p.493.

54. Opton, E.M., Jr., Letter to the members of the panel, National Institute of Health Consensus Development Conference on Electroconvulsive Therapy, June 4, 1985, as cited in Frank, L.R., "Electroshock: death, brain damage, memory loss, and brainwashing," *op. cit.*, p. 497.

55. Boodman, S.G., "Shock therapy . . . it's back," *op cit.*

56. Cauchon, Dennis, "Patients often aren't informed of full danger," *op. cit.*

57. Frank, L.R., "Electroshock: death, brain damage, memory loss, and brainwashing," *op. cit.*, p.494.

58. *Ibid.*

59. Viscott, D., *The Making of a Psychiatrist*. Greenwich, CT, Faucett, 1972, in Leonard Roy Frank, "Electroshock: Death . . ." *op. cit.*, p.494

CHAPTER FOUR

1. Journal of the American Medical Association, August 2001.

2. 346 The New England Journal of Medicine, Feb 14, 2002, pp.498–505, 524–531.

6. Boseley S, Scandal of scientists who take money for papers ghostwritten by drug companies, The Guardian, February 7, 2002.

7. Is academic medicine for sale?, 342(20), N Engl J Med, May 18, 2000, pp.1516–8.

8. Postapproval Risks 1976–1985, GAO/PEMD 90–15 FDA DRUG Review, p.3)

5. Drugmaker Upset: New book attacks popular antidepressant Prozac, Associated Press, April 6, 2000.

6. Glenmullen J, Prozac Backlash.

7. Kramer P, Listening to Prozac.

8. Breggin, Peter R, M.D., Your Drug May Be Your Problem: How and Why to

References

Stop Taking Psychiatric Medications, Perseus Books, 1999.

9. Breggin, Peter R, M.D., Talking Back to Ritalin, Revised : What Doctors Aren't Telling You About Stimulants and ADHD, Perseus Books, 2001.

10. Breggin, Peter R, M.D., Toxic Psychiatry: Why therapy, empathy, and love must replace the drugs, electroshock, and biochemical theories of the "new psychiatry", St. Martin's Press, 1994.

11. Breggin, Peter R, M.D., The Anti-Depressant Fact Book: What Your Doctor Won't Tell You About Prozac, Zoloft, Paxil, Celexa and Luvox.

12. Breggin, Peter R, M.D., Talking Back to Prozac: What doctors aren't telling you about today's most controversial drug, St. Martin's Press, 1995.

13. Breggin, Peter R, M.D., Brain-Disabling Treatments in Psychiatry: Drugs, Electroshock, and the Role of the FDA, Springer Publishing Co., 1997.

14. *http://www.breggin.com/*

15. Breggin, Peter R, M.D., Electroshock: Its Brain-Disabling Effects, Springer Publishing Company, 1979.

16. *http://www.breggin.com/*

17. Mansbridge P, CBC News and Current Affairs, Jun 12, 2001.

18. Paxil Maker Ordered to Pay $8 Million, The Associated Press, June 6, 2002.

20. Wang PN, Liao SQ, Liu RS, Liu CY, Chao HT, Lu SR, Yu HY, Wang SJ, Liu HC, Effects of estrogen on cognition, mood, and cerebral blood flow in Alzheimer's Disease: a controlled study, 54(11) Neurology, June 13, 2000, pp.2061–6.

21. Breuer B, Martucci C, Wallenstein S, Likourezos A, Libow LS, Peterson A, Zumoff B, Relationship of endogenous levels of sex hormones to cognition and depression in frail, elderly women, 10(3) Am J Geriatr Psychiatry, May 2002, pp.311–20.

22. Campbell M, Silva RR, Kafantaris V, Locascio JJ, Gonzalez NM, Lee D, Lynch NS, Predictors of side effects associated with lithium administration in children, 27(3) Psychopharmacol Bull., 1991, pp.373–80.

23. Silva RR, Campbell M, Golden RR, Small AM, Pataki CS, Rosenberg CR, Side effects associated with lithium and placebo administration in aggressive children, 28(3) Psychopharmacol Bull., 1992, pp.319–26.

24. Malone RP, Delaney MA, Luebbert JF, Cater J, Campbell M, A double-blind placebo-controlled study of lithium in hospitalized aggressive children and adolescents with conduct disorder, 57(7) Arch Gen Psychiatry, July 2000, pp.649–54.

25. Mavissakalian M, Perel J, Guo S, Specific side effects of long-term

References

imipramine management of panic disorder, 22(2) J Clin Psychopharmacol, Apr 2002, pp.155–61.

26. ten Holt WL, van Iperen CE, Schrijver G, Bartelink AK, Severe hyponatremia during therapy with fluoxetine, 156(6) Arch Intern Med., Mar 25, 1996, pp.681–2.

27. Girault C, Richard JC, Chevron V, Goulle JP, Droy JM, Bonmarchand G, Leroy J, Syndrome of inappropriate secretion of antidiuretic hormone in two elderly women with elevated serum fluoxetine, 35(1) J Toxicol Clin Toxicol, 1997, pp.93–5.

28. Burke D, Fanker S, Fluoxetine and the syndrome of inappropriate secretion of antidiuretic hormone (SIADH), 30(2) Aust N Z J Psychiatry, Apr 1996, pp.295–8.

29. Bourguignon RP, Dangers of fluoxetine, 349(9046) Lancet, Jan 18, 1997, p.214.

30. Braun D, Nippert B, Loeuille D, Blain H, Trechot P, Interstitial pneumopathy induced by fluoxetine, 20(10) Rev Med Interne, Oct 1999, pp.949–50.

31. Martinez Ortiz JJ, Hyperthyroidism secondary to antidepressive treatment with fluoxetine, 16(11) An Med Interna, Nov 1999, pp.583–4.

32. Bates GD, Khin-Maung-Zaw F., Movement disorder with fluoxetine, 37(1) J Am Acad Child Adolesc Psychiatry, Jan 1998, pp.14–5.

33. Wilmshurst PT, Kumar AV, Subhyaloid haemorrhage with fluoxetine, 10(Pt 1) Eye, 1996, p.141.

34. Michael A, Mayer C, Fluoxetine-induced anaesthesia of vagina and nipples, 176 Br J Psychiatry, Mar 2000, p.299.

35. Hwang AS, Magraw RM, Syndrome of inappropriate secretion of antidiuretic hormone due to fluoxetine, 146(3) Am J Psychiatry, Mar 1989, p.399.

36. Anand KS, Prasad A, Pradhan SC, Biswas A, Fluoxetine-induced tremors, 47(6) J Assoc Physicians India, June 1999, pp.651–2.

37. Cohen BJ, Mahelsky M, Adler L, More cases of SIADH with fluoxetine, 147(7) Am J Psychiatry, July 1990, pp.948–9.

38. Vishwanath BM, Navalgund AA, Cusano W, Navalgund KA, Fluoxetine as a cause of SIADH, 148(4) Am J Psychiatry, April 1991, pp.542–3.

39. Buchman N, Strous RD, Baruch Y, Side effects of long-term treatment with fluoxetine, 25(1) Clin Neuropharmacol, Jan 2002, pp.55–7.

40. Stanford JA, Currier TD, Gerhardt GA, Acute locomotor effects of fluoxetine, sertraline, and nomifensine in young versus aged Fischer 344 rats,

References

71(1–2) Pharmacol Biochem Behav, Jan-Feb 2002, pp.325–32.

41. Rothschild AJ, Sexual side effects of antidepressants, 61 Suppl 11 J Clin Psychiatry, 2000, pp.28–36.
42. Balon R, Yeragani VK, Pohl R, Ramesh C, Sexual dysfunction during antidepressant treatment, 54(6) J Clin Psychiatry, June 1993, pp.209–12.
43. Opbroek A, Delgado PL, Laukes C, McGahuey C, Katsanis J, Moreno FA, Manber R, Emotional blunting associated with SSRI-induced sexual dysfunction. Do SSRIs inhibit emotional responses?, 5(2) Int J Neuropsychopharmacol, June 2002, pp.147–51.
44. Murray JB, Physiological mechanisms of sexual dysfunction side effects associated with antidepressant medication, 132(4) J Psychol, July 1998, pp.407–16.
45. Woodrum ST, Brown CS, Management of SSRI-induced sexual dysfunction, 32(11) Ann Pharmacother, Nov 1998, pp.1209–15.
46. Sproule BA, Naranjo CA, Brenmer KE, Hassan PC, Selective serotonin reuptake inhibitors and CNS drug interactions. A critical review of the evidence, 33(6) Clin Pharmacokinet, Dec 1997, pp.454–71.
47. Bozikas V, Petrikis P, Karavatos A, Urinary retention caused after fluoxetine-risperidone combination, 15(2) J Psychopharmacol, June 2001, pp.142–3.
48. Fava M, Rankin M, Sexual functioning and SSRIs, 63 Suppl 5 J Clin Psychiatry, 2002, pp.13–6.
49. Bagdy G, Graf M, Anheuer ZE, Modos EA, Kantor S, Anxiety-like effects induced by acute fluoxetine, sertraline or m-CPP treatment are reversed by pretreatment with the 5–HT2C receptor antagonist SB-242084 but not the 5–HT1A receptor antagonist WAY-100635, 4(4) Int J Neuropsychopharmacol, Dec 2001, pp.399–408.
50. Nurnberg HG, Lauriello J, Hensley PL, Parker LM, Keith SJ, Sildenafil for iatrogenic serotonergic antidepressant medication-induced sexual dysfunction in 4 patients, 60(1) J Clin Psychiatry, Jan 1999, pp.33–5.
51. Tollefson GD, Sayler ME, Course of psychomotor agitation during pharmacotherapy of depression: analysis from double-blind controlled trials with fluoxetine, 4(6) Depress Anxiety, 1996, pp.294–311.
52. Reichenberg-Ullman J, Homeopathy: a highly effective alternative to antidepressants (for treatment of mental depression), Townsend Letter for Doctors and Patients, April 2001.
53. Montgomery SA, Judge R, Treatment of depression with associated anxiety:

References

comparisons of tricyclic antidepressants and selective serotonin reuptake inhibitors, 403 Acta Psychiatr Scand Suppl, 2000, pp.9–16.

54. Cook BL, Helms PM, Smith RE, Tsai M, Unipolar depression in the elderly. Reoccurrence on discontinuation of tricyclic antidepressants, 10(2) J Affect Disord, Mar 1986, pp.91–4.

55. Graber MA, Weckmann M, Pharmaceutical company internet sites as sources of information about antidepressant medications, 16(6) CNS Drugs, 2002, pp.419–23.

56. Anderson JL, The immune system and major depression, 6(2) Adv Neuroimmunol, 1996, pp.119–29.

57. Maes M, Vandoolaeghe E, Ranjan R, Bosmans E, Bergmans R, Desnyder R, Increased serum interleukin-1–receptor-antagonist concentrations in major depression, 36(1–2) J Affect Disorder, Dec 24, 1995, pp.29–36.

58. Elgun S, Keskinege A, Kumbasar H, Dipeptidyl peptidase IV and adenosine deaminase activity. Decrease in depression, 24(8) Psychoneuroendocrinology, Nov 1999, pp.823–32.

59. Irwin M, Psychoneuroimmunology of depression: clinical implications, 16(1) Brain Behav Immun, Feb 2002, pp.1–16.

60. Hese RT, Gruszczynski W, Szwed A, Kielc M, Zalitacz M, Comparative studies of adverse effects in patients with refractory depression treated with amitryptyline, mianserin and unilateral ECT, 35(2) Psychiatr Pol, Mar-Apr 2001, pp. 219–29.

61. Clayton AH, Pradko JF, Croft HA, Montano CB, Leadbetter RA, Bolden-Watson C, Bass KI, Donahue RM, Jamerson BD, Metz A., Prevalence of sexual dysfunction among newer antidepressants, 63(4) J Clin Psychiatry, Apr 2002, pp.357–66.

62. Lemmo Walter, Unraveling antidepressant medications: what you & your physician may not know, Townsend Letter for Doctors and Patients, July 2001.

63. Covelli V, Maffione AB, Nacci C, Tato E., Jirillo E, Stress, neuropsychiatric disorders and immunological effects exerted by benzodiazepines, 20(2) Immunopharmacol Immunotoxicol, May 1998, pp.199–209.

64. Kupfer DJ, Pathophysiology and management of insomnia during depression, 11(4) Ann Clin Psychiatry, Dec 1999, pp.267–76.

65. Miller NS, Gold MS, Benzodiazepines: a major problem. Introduction, 8(1–2) J Subst Abuse Treat, 1991, pp.3–7.

66. Juergens SM, Benzodiazepines and addiction, 16(1) Psychiatr Clin North

References

Am, March 1993, pp.75–86.

67. Holden J, Benzodiazepine dependence, 233(1478) Practitioner, Nov 8, 1989, pp.1479–80, 1483.

68. Bernik MA, Soares MB, Soares CN, Benzodiazepines: patterns of use, tolerance and dependence, 48(1) Arq Neuropsiquiatr, Mar 1990, pp.131–7.

69. Olivier H, Fitz-Gerald MJ, Babiak B., Benzodiazepines revisited, 150(10) J La State Med Soc, Oct 1998, pp.483–5.

70. Kuribara H, Kishi E, Maruyama Y, Does dihydrohonokiol, a potent anxiolytic compound, result in the development of benzodiazepine-like side effects?, 52(8) J Pharm Pharmacol, Aug 2000, pp.1017–22.

71. Pettinati HM, Stephens SM, Willis KM, Robin SE, Evidence for less improvement in depression in patients taking benzodiazepines during unilateral ECT, 147(8) Am J Psychiatry, Aug 1990, 1029–35.

72. Simmer ED, A fugue-like state associated with diazepam use, 164(6) Mil Med, June 1999, pp.442–3.

73. Engel WR, Grau A, Inappropriate secretion of antidiuretic hormone associated with lorazepam, 297(6652) BMJ, Oct 1 1988, p.858.

74. Loo H, Olie JP, Poirier MF, Amado I, Psychotropic Drugs and Behavior, 56(2) Ann Pharm Fr, 1998, pp.75–82.

75. Paterniti S, Dufouil C, Alperovitch A., Long-term benzodiazepine use and cognitive decline in the elderly: the Epidemiology of Vascular Aging Study, 22(3) J Clin Psychopharmacol, Jun 2002, pp.285–93.

76. Pigott TA, Seay SM, A review of the efficacy of selective serotonin reuptake inhibitors in obsessive-compulsive disorder, 60(2) J Clin Psychiatry, Feb 1999, pp.101–16.

77. Papakostas Y, Stefanis C, Sinouri A, Trikkas G, Papadimitriou G, Pittoulis S., Increases in prolactin levels following bilateral and unilateral ECT, 141(12) Am J Psychiatry, Dec 1984, pp.1623–4.

78. Markowitz JS, Kellner CH, DeVane CL, Beale MD, Folk J, Burns C, Liston HL, Intranasal sumatriptan in post-ECT headache: results of an open-label trial, 17(4) J ECT, Dec 2001, pp.280–3.

79. Brodaty H, Hickie I, Mason C, Prenter L, A prospective follow-up study of ECT outcome in older depressed patients, 60(2) J Affect Disord, Nov 2000, pp.101–11.

80. Fromm-Auch D, Comparison of unilateral and bilateral ECT: evidence for selective memory impairment, 141 Br J Psychiatry, Dec 1982, pp.608–13.

81. Squire LR, Zouzounis JA, ECT and memory: brief pulse versus sine wave,

143(5), Am J Psychiatry, May 1986, pp.596–601.

82. Pettinati HM, Rosenberg J, Memory self-ratings before and after electro-convulsive therapy: depression-versus ECT induced, 19(4) Biol Psychiatry, Apr 1984, pp.539–48.

83. Calev A, Nigal D, Shapira B, Tubi N, Chazan S, Ben-Yehuda Y, Kugelmass S, Lerer B, Early and long-term effects of electroconvulsive therapy and depression on memory and other cognitive functions, 179(9) J Nerv Ment Dis, Sep 1991, pp.526–33.

84. Squire LB, Chace PM, Slater PC, Retrograde amnesia following electro-convulsive therapy, 260(5554) Nature, Apr 29, 1976, pp.775–7.

85. Frith CD, Stevens M, Johnstone EC, Deakin JF, Lawler P, Crow TJ, Effects of ECT and depression on various aspects of memory, 142 Br J Psychiatry, June 1983, pp.610–7.

86. McAllister DA, Perri MG, Jordan RC, Rauscher FP, Sattin A, Effects of ECT given two vs. three times weekly, 21(1) Psychiatry Res, May 1987, pp.63–9.

87. Stewart C, Jeffery K, Reid I, LTP-like synaptic efficacy changes following electroconvulsive stimulation, 5(9) Neuroreport, May 9, 1994, pp.1041–4.

88. Calev A, Cohen R, Tubi N, Nigal D, Shapira B, Kugelmass S, Lerer B, Dis-orientation and Bilateral Moderately Suprathreshold Titrated ECT, 7(2) Convuls Ther 1991, pp.99–110.

89. Neylan TC, Canick JD, Hall SE, Reus VI, Sapolsky RM, Wolkowitz OM, Cortisol levels predict cognitive impairment induced by electroconvulsive therapy, 50(5) Biol Psychiatry, Sep 1, 2001, pp.331–6.

90. Tang WK, Ungvari GS, Asystole during electroconvulsive therapy: a case report, 35(3) Aust N Z J Psychiatry, Jun 2001, pp.382–5.

91. Ng C, Schweitzer I, Alexopoulos P, Celi E, Wong L, Tuckwell V, Sergejew A, Tiller J, Efficacy and cognitive effects of right unilateral electroconvul-sive therapy, 16(4) J ECT, Dec 2000, pp.370–9.

92. Dubovsky SL, Buzan R, Thomas M, Kassner C, Cullum CM, Nicardipine improves the antidepressant action of ECT but does not improve cognition, 17(1) J ECT, Mar 2001, pp.3–10.

93. Rao V, Lyketsos CG, The benefits and risks of ECT for patients with pri-mary dementia who also suffer from depression, 15(8) Int J Geriatr Psychi-atry, Aug 2000, pp.729–35.

94. Lisanby SH, Maddox JH, Prudic J, Devanand DP, Sackeim HA, The

effects of electroconvulsive therapy on memory of autobiographical and public events, 57(6) Arch Gen Psychiatry, Jun 2000, pp.581–90.

95. Shapira B, Tubi N, Lerer B, Balancing speed of response to ECT in major depression and adverse cognitive effects: role of treatment schedule, 16(2) J ECT, Jun 2000, pp.97–109.

96. Sackeim HA, Luber B, Moeller JR, Prudic J, Devanand DP, Nobler MS, Electrophysiological correlates of the adverse cognitive effects of electroconvulsive therapy, 16(2) J ECT, Jun 2000, pp.110–20.

97. Squire LR, Slater PC, Miller PL, Retrograde amnesia and bilateral electroconvulsive therapy. Long-term follow-up, 38(1) Arch Gen Psychiatry, Jan 1981, pp.89–95.

98. Shellenberger W, Miller MJ, Small IF, Milstein V, Stout JR, Follow-up study of memory deficits after ECT, 27(4) Can J Psychiatry, Jun 1982, pp.325–9.

99. Sobin C, Sackeim HA, Prudic J, Devanand DP, Moody BJ, McElhiney MC, Predictors of retrograde amnesia following ECT, 152(7) Am J Psychiatry, Jul 1995, pp.995–1001.

100. Weiner RD, Retrograde amnesia with electroconvulsive therapy: characteristics and implications, 57(6) Arch Gen Psychiatry, Jun 2000, pp.591–2.

101. Rosenberg J, Pettinati HM, Differential memory complaints after bilateral and unilateral ECT, 141(9) Am J Psychiatry, Sep 1984, pp.1071–4.

CHAPTER FIVE

1a. Epidemiology of medical error. Weingart, SN. et al. BMJ 2000;320: 774–777 (18 March).

2a. Reporting and preventing medical mishaps: lessons from non-medical near miss reporting systems. Barach, P. and Small S. BMJ 2000;320:759–763 (18 March).

3a. The scandal of poor medical research. Altman, DG. BMJ 1994; 308:283–284 (29 January).

4a. Sponsored drug trials show more-favourable outcomes. Wahlbeck K, et al. BMJ 1999;318:464 (13 February).

5a. Physicians and the Pharmaceutical Industry: Is a Gift Ever Just a Gift? Wazana, A. JAMA 2000;283:373–380.

6a. Reasons for not seeing drug representatives. Griffith D. BMJ 1999;319·

References

69–70 (10 July).

7a. Medical societies accused of being beholden to the drugs industry. Gottlieb S. BMJ 1999;319:1321 (20 November).

8a. "Routine" preoperative studies. Which studies in which patients? Marcello PW, Roberts PL. Surg Clin North Am 1996 Feb;76(1):11–23.

9a. Value of routine preoperative chest x-rays: a meta-analysis. Archer C, Levy AR, McGregor M. Can J Anaesth 1993 Nov;40(11):1022–7.

10a. Accuracy of fecal occult blood screening for colorectal neoplasia A prospective study using Hemoccult and HemoQuant tests. Ahlquist DA, et al. JAMA 1993 Mar 10;269(10):1262–7.

11a. Consumption of NSAIDs and the development of congestive heart failure in elderly patients: an underrecognized public health problem. Page J, Henry D. Arch Intern Med 2000 Mar 27;160(6):777–84.

12a. Study throws doubt on protective effects of HRT for heart disease. Gottlieb S. BMJ 2000;320:826 (25 March).

13a. Impact of postmenopausal hormone therapy on cardiovascular events and cancer: pooled data from clinical trials. Elina Hemminki, et al. BMJ 1997;315:149–153 (19 July).

14a. Mortality associated with oral contraceptive use 25 year follow up of cohort of 46 000 women from Royal College of General Practitioners' oral contraception study. Beral V, et al. BMJ 1999;318:96–100 (9 January).

15a. Oral contraceptives and fatal pulmonary embolism. Parkin L, Skegg DCG, Wilson M, Herbison GP, Paul C. Lancet 2000; 355: 2088,2133–2134.

16a. Ovarian tumors in a cohort of infertile women. Rossing MA, Daling JR, Weiss NS, Moore DE, Self SG. N Engl J Med 1994 Sep 22;331(12): 771–6.

17a. Rates of Cesarean delivery—United States, 1993. MMWR Morb Mortal Wkly Rep 1995 Apr 21;44(15):303–7.

18a. Cesarean section: medical benefits and costs. Shearer EL. Soc Sci Med 1993 Nov;37(10):1223–31.

19a. Drug use and pulmonary death rates in increasingly symptomatic asthma patients in the UK. Meier CR; Jick H. Thorax, 52(7):612–7 1997 Jul

20a. Adverse effects of inhaled corticosteroids. Hanania NA; Chapman KR; Kesten S. Am J Med, 98(2):196–208 1995 Feb

21a. Cancer undefeated. Bailar JC 3rd; Gornik HL. N Engl J Med, 336(22):1569–74 1997 May 29.

22a. Gallbladder carcinoma: a 28 year experience. Frezza EE, Mezghebe H. Int

References

Surg 1997 Jul-Sep;82(3):295–300.

23a. Pathological prognostic factors in the second British Stomach Cancer Group trial of adjuvant therapy in resectable gastric cancer. Yu CC; et al. J Cancer, 71(5):1106–10 1995 May.

24a. Pre-operative radiotherapy prolongs survival in operable esophageal carcinoma: a randomized, multicenter study of pre-operative radiotherapy and chemotherapy The second Scandinavian trial in esophageal cancer. Nygaard K; et al. World J Surg, 16(6):1104–9; discussion 1110 1992 Nov-Dec.

25a. Lack of evidence for a role of chemotherapy in the routine management of locally advanced head and neck cancer. Tannock IF; Browman G. J Clin Oncol, 4(7):1121–6 1986 Jul.

26a. Outcome of combination chemotherapy in extensive stage small-cell lung cancer: any treatment related progress? Lassen UN, Hirsch FR, Osterlind K, Bergman B, Dombernowsky P. Lung Cancer 1998 Jun;20(3):151–60

27a. Interferon alfa-2a and interleukin-2 with or without cisplatin in metastatic melanoma: a randomized trial of the European Organization for Research and Treatment of Cancer Melanoma Cooperative Group. Keilholz U; et al. J Clin Oncol, 15(7):2579–88 1997 Jul.

28a. Randomized study of 5–FU and CCNU in pancreatic cancer Report of the Veterans Administration Surgical Adjuvant Cancer Chemotherapy Study Group. Frey C; Twomey P; Keehn R; Elliott D; Higgins G. Cancer, 47(1):27–31 1981 Jan 1.

29a. Failure of cytotoxic chemotherapy, 1983–1988, and the emerging role of monoclonal antibodies for renal cancer. Yagoda A; Bander NH. Urol Int, 44(6):338–45 1989.

30a. Late effects of radiation therapy for cancer of the uterine cervix. Zippin C; Lum D; Kohn HI; Bailar JC 3d. Cancer Detect Prev, 4(1–4):487–92 1981.

31a. Intensive blood-glucose control with sulphonylureas or insulin compared with conventional treatment and risk of complications in patients with type 2 diabetes (UKPDS 33). UK Prospective Diabetes Study (UKPDS) Group. Lancet 1998 Sep 12;352(9131):837–53

32a. Controversies in Management: Case for early treatment is not established. Chadwick, D. BMJ 1995;310:177–178 (21 January).

33a. Notice to Readers: Fourth Decennial International Conference on Nosocomial and Healthcare-Associated Infections. MMWR, February 25, 2000 / 49(07);138.

References

CONCLUSION

1. Luo H, Meng F, Jia Y, Zhao X. Clinical research on the therapeutic effect of the electro-acupuncture treatment in patients with depression. *Psychiatry Clin Neurosci*. 1998 Dec;52 Suppl:S338–40.

2. Roschke J, Wolf C, Muller MJ, Wagner P, Mann K, Grozinger M, Bech S.The benefit from whole body acupuncture in major depression. *J Affect Disord*. 2000 Jan-Mar;57(1–3):73–81.

3. Knight B, Mudge C, Openshaw S, White A, Hart A.Effect of acupuncture on nausea of pregnancy: a randomized, controlled trial. *Obstet Gynecol*. 2001 Feb;97(2):184–8.

4. Eich H, Agelink MW, Lehmann E, Lemmer W, Klieser E. Acupuncture in patients with minor depressive episodes and generalized anxiety. Results of an experimental study. *Fortschr Neurol Psychiatr*. 2000 Mar;68(3):137–44.

5. Bullock ML, Kiresuk TJ, Sherman RE, Lenz SK, Culliton PD, Boucher TA, Nolan CJ. A large randomized placebo controlled study of auricular acupuncture for alcohol dependence. *J Subst Abuse Treat*. 2002 Mar; 22(2):71–7.

6. Russell AL, McCarty MF. DL-phenylalanine markedly potentiates opiate analgesia–an example of nutrient/pharmaceutical up-regulation of the endogenous analgesia system. *Med Hypotheses*. 2000 Oct;55(4):283–8.

7. Ernst E. A primer of complementary and alternative medicine commonly used by cancer patients. *Med J Aust*. 2001 Jan 15;174(2):88–92.

8. Manber R, Allen JJ, Morris MM. Alternative treatments for depression: empirical support and relevance to women. *J Clin Psychiatry*. 2002 Jul;63(7):628–40.

9. Dello Buono M, Urciuoli O, Marietta P, Padoani W, De Leo D. Alternative medicine in a sample of 655 community-dwelling elderly. *J Psychosom Res*. 2001 Mar;50(3):147–54.

10. Ernst E. A primer of complementary and alternative medicine commonly used by cancer patients. *Med J Aust*. 2001 Jan 15;174(2):88–92.

11. d'Elia G, Hanson L, Raotma H. L-tryptophan and 5–hydroxytryptophan in the treatment of depression. A review. *Acta Psychiatr Scand*. 1978 Mar;57(3):239–52.

12. Lam RW, Zis AP, Grewal A, Delgado PL, Charney DS, Krystal JH. Effects of rapid tryptophan depletion in patients with seasonal affective disorder in remission after light therapy. *Arch Gen Psychiatry*. 1996 Jan;53(1):41–4.

13. Abou-Saleh MT, Ghubash R, Karim L, Krymski M, Anderson DN. The role

References

of pterins and related factors in the biology of early postpartum depression. *Eur Neuropsychopharmacol*. 1999 Jun;9(4):295–300.

14. Spillmann MK, Van der Does AJ, Rankin MA, Vuolo RD, Alpert JE, Nierenberg AA, Rosenbaum JF, Hayden D, Schoenfeld D, Fava M. Tryptophan depletion in SSRI-recovered depressed outpatients. *Psychopharmacology (Berl)*. 2001 May;155(2):123–7.

15. Blokland A, Lieben C, Deutz NE. Anxiogenic and depressive-like effects, but no cognitive deficits, after repeated moderate tryptophan depletion in the rat. *J Psychopharmacol*. 2002 Mar;16(1):39–49.

16. Young SN, Leyton M. The role of serotonin in human mood and social interaction. Insight from altered tryptophan levels. *Pharmacol Biochem Behav*. 2002 Apr;71(4):857–65.

17. Khalsa DS. Integrated medicine and the prevention and reversal of memory loss. *Altern Ther Health Med* (1998 Nov) 4(6):38–43.

18. Holmes C, Hopkins V, Hensford C, MacLaughlin V, Wilkinson D, Rosenvinge H. Lavender oil as a treatment for agitated behaviour in severe dementia: a placebo controlled study. *Int J Geriatr Psychiatry*. 2002 Apr;17(4):305–8.

19. Dunn C, Sleep J, Collett D. Sensing an improvement: an experimental study to evaluate the use of aromatherapy, massage and periods of rest in an intensive care unit. *J Adv Nurs*. 1995 Jan;21(1):34–40.

20. Burns E, Blamey C, Ersser SJ, Lloyd AJ, Barnetson L. The use of aromatherapy in intrapartum midwifery practice an observational study. *Complement Ther Nurs Midwifery*. 2000 Feb;6(1):33–4.

21. Buckle J. The role of aromatherapy in nursing care. *Nurs Clin North Am*. 2001 Mar;36(1):57–72.

22. Lee KG, Mitchell A, Shibamoto T. Antioxidative activities of aroma extracts isolated from natural plants. *Biofactors*. 2000;13(1–4):173–8.

23. Bhattacharya SK, Battacharya A, Sairam K, Ghosal S. Anxiolytic-antidepressant activity of Withania somnifera glycowithanolides: an experimental study. *Phytomedicine*. 2000 Dec;7(6):463–9.

24. Bhattacharya SK, Battacharya A, Chakrabarti A. Adaptogenic activity of Siotone, a polyherbal formulation of Ayurvedic rasayanas. *Indian J Exp Biol*. 2000 Feb;38(2):119–28.

25. Jaiswal AK, Bhattacharya SK, Acharya SB. Anxiolytic activity of Azadirachta indica leaf extract in rats. *Indian J Exp Biol*. 1994 Jul;32(7):489–91.

26. Long L, Huntley A, Ernst E. Which complementary and alternative therapies benefit which conditions? A survey of the opinions of 223 professional

References

organizations. *Complement Ther Med* 2001 Sep;9(3):178–85

27. Saeki Y. The effect of foot-bath with or without the essential oil of lavender on the autonomic nervous system: a randomized trial. *Complement Ther Med.* 2000 Mar;8(1):2–7.

28. Rastelli A, Sartori A, Ferrari G. Arsenic-iron balneotherapy in anxiety syndromes. Controlled clinical study at the Levico thermal baths. *Minerva Med.* 1985 Dec 22;76(49–50):2291–301.

29. Evcik D, Kizilay B, Gokcen E. The effects of balneotherapy on fibromyalgia patients. *Rheumatol Int.* 2002 Jun;22(2):56–9.

30. Armijo Valenzuela M. Spa therapy and sadness. *An R Acad Nac Med (Madr).* 1999;116(2):279–95.

31. Buskila D, Abu-Shakra M, Neumann L, Odes L, Shneider E, Flusser D, Sukenik S. Balneotherapy for fibromyalgia at the Dead Sea. *Rheumatol Int.* 2001 Apr;20(3):105–8.

32. Wright J, Clum GA, Roodman A, Febbraro GA. A bibliotherapy approach to relapse prevention in individuals with panic attacks. *J Anxiety Disord.* 2000 Sep-Oct;14(5):483–99.

33. Christensen H, Griffiths KM, Korten A. Web-based cognitive behavior therapy: analysis of site usage and changes in depression and anxiety scores. *J Med Internet Res* 2002 Jan-Mar;4(1):e3.

34. Kupshik GA, Fisher CR. Assisted bibliotherapy: effective, efficient treatment for moderate anxiety problems. *Br J Gen Pract.* 1999 Jan;49(438):47–8.

35. Montgomery P. Media-based behavioural treatments for behavioural disorders in children. *Cochrane Database Syst Rev.* 2001;(2):CD002206.

36. Pearlstein T, Steiner M. Non-antidepressant treatment of premenstrual syndrome. *J Clin Psychiatry.* 2000;61 Suppl 12:22–7.

37. Bauman WA, Shaw S, Jayatilleke E, Spungen AM, Herbert V. Increased intake of calcium reverses vitamin B12 malabsorption induced by metformin. *Diabetes Care.* 2000 Sep;23(9):1227–31.

38. Mercola J. Low cholesterol causes aggressive behavior and depression. *Townsend Letter for Doctors and Patients.* 2001 May.

39. Heimberg RG. Cognitive-behavioral therapy for social anxiety disorder: current status and future directions. *Biol Psychiatry* 2002 Jan 1;51(1):101–8.

40. Clark DB, Agras WS. The assessment and treatment of performance anxiety in musicians. *Am J Psychiatry.* 1991 May;148(5):598–605.

41. Generalised anxiety disorder: treatment options. Sramek JJ, Zarotsky V, Cutler NR. *Drugs.* 2002;62(11):1635–48.

References

42. Safren SA, Heimberg RG, Brown EJ, Holle C. Quality of life in social phobia. *Depress Anxiety* 1996–97;4(3):126–33.

43. Pearlstein T, Steiner M. Non-antidepressant treatment of premenstrual syndrome. *J Clin Psychiatry*. 2000;61 Suppl 12:22–7.

44. Goisman RM, Warshaw MG, Keller MB. Psychosocial treatment prescriptions for generalized anxiety disorder, panic disorder, and social phobia, 1991–1996. *Am J Psychiatry*. 1999 Nov;156(11):1819–21.

45. Demeter E, Rihmer Z, Frecska E. Colour associations as predictors of the effectiveness of anti-depressant pharmacotherapy in endogenous depressive patients. *Psychopathology*. 1985;18(5–6):305–9.

46. de Craen AJ, Roos PJ, Leonard de Vries A, Kleijnen J. Effect of colour of drugs: systematic review of perceived effect of drugs and of their effectiveness. *BMJ*. 1996 Dec 21–28;313(7072):1624–6.

47. Coldwell SE, Getz T, Milgrom P, Prall CW, Spadafora A, Ramsay DS. CARL: a LabVIEW 3 computer program for conducting exposure therapy for the treatment of dental injection fear. *Behav Res Ther*. 1998 Apr;36(4):429–41.

48. Arlt W, Callies F, Allolio B. DHEA replacement in women with adrenal insufficiency—pharmacokinetics, bioconversion and clinical effects on well-being, sexuality and cognition. *Endocr Res*. 2000 Nov;26(4):505–11.

49. Cogan E. DHEA: orthodox or alternative medicine? *Rev Med Brux*. 2001 Sep;22(4):A381–6.

50. Young AH, Gallagher P, Porter RJ. Elevation of the cortisol-dehydroepiandrosterone ratio in drug-free depressed patients. *Am J Psychiatry*. 2002 Jul;159(7):1237–9.

51. Goodyer IM, Herbert J, Tamplin A, Altham PM. First-episode major depression in adolescents. Affective, cognitive and endocrine characteristics of risk status and predictors of onset. *Br J Psychiatry*. 2000 Feb;176:142–9.

52. Nagata C, Shimizu H, Takami R, Hayashi M, Takeda N, Yasuda K. Serum concentrations of estradiol and dehydroepiandrosterone sulfate and soy product intake in relation to psychologic well-being in peri- and postmenopausal Japanese women. *Metabolism*. 2000 Dec;49(12):1561–4.

53. Michael A, Jenaway A, Paykel ES, Herbert J. Altered salivary dehydroepiandrosterone levels in major depression in adults. *Biol Psychiatry*. 2000 Nov 15;48(10):989–95.

54. Fabian TJ, Dew MA, Pollock BG, Reynolds CF 3rd, Mulsant BH, Butters MA, Zmuda MD, Linares AM, Trottini M, Kroboth PD. Endogenous con-

References

centrations of DHEA and DHEA-S decrease with remission of depression in older adults. *Biol Psychiatry*. 2001 Nov 15;50(10):767–74.

55. Huppert FA, Van Niekerk JK, Herbert J. Dehydroepiandrosterone (DHEA) supplementation for cognition and well-being. *Cochrane Database Syst Rev*. 2000;(2):CD000304.

56. Cohen JH, Kristal AR, Neumark-Sztainaer D, Rock CL, Neuhouser ML. Psychological distress is associated with unhealthful dietary practices. *J Am Diet Assoc*. 2002 May;102(5):699–703.

57. Balcombe NR, Ferry PG, Saweirs WM. Nutritional status and well being. Is there a relationship between body mass index and the well-being of older people? *Curr Med Res Opin*. 2001;17(1):1–7.

58. Schmidt MH, Mocks P, Lay B, Eisert HG, Fojkar R, Fritz-Sigmund D, Marcus A, Musaeus B. Does oligoantigenic diet influence hyperactive/conduct-disordered children—a controlled trial. *Eur Child Adolesc Psychiatry*. 1997 Jun;6(2):88–95.

59. Vatn MH. Food intolerance and psychosomatic experience. *Scand J Work Environ Health*. 1997;23 Suppl 3:75–8.

60. Rogers PJ. A healthy body, a healthy mind: long-term impact of diet on mood and cognitive function. *Proc Nutr Soc*. 2001 Feb;60(1):135–43.

61. Breakey J. The role of diet and behaviour in childhood. *J Paediatr Child Health*. 1997 Jun;33(3):190–4.

62. Bittman BB, Berk LS, Felten DL, Westengard J, Simonton OC, Pappas J, Ninehouser M. Composite effects of group drumming music therapy on modulation of neuroendocrine-immune parameters in normal subjects. *Altern Ther Health Med*. 2001 Jan;7(1):38–47.

63. Horrobin DF. The role of essential fatty acids and prostaglandins in the premenstrual syndrome. *J Reprod Med*. 1983 Jul;28(7):465–8.

64. Stoll AL, Severus WE, Freeman MP, Rueter S, Zboyan HA, Diamond E, Cress KK, Marangell LB. Omega 3 fatty acids in bipolar disorder: a preliminary double-blind, placebo-controlled trial. *Arch Gen Psychiatry*. 1999 May;56(5):407–12.

65. Rudin DO. The major psychoses and neuroses as omega-3 essential fatty acid deficiency syndrome: substrate pellagra. *Biol Psychiatry*. 1981 Sep;16(9):837–50.

66. Mischoulon D, Fava M. Docosahexanoic acid and omega-3 fatty acids in depression. *Psychiatr Clin North Am*. 2000 Dec;23(4):785–94.

References

67. Martinsen EW. Physical activity for mental health. *Tidsskr Nor Laegeforen.* 2000 Oct 20;120(25):3054–6.
68. Jorm AF, Christensen H, Griffiths KM, Rodgers B. Effectiveness of complementary and self-help treatments for depression. *Med J Aust.* 2002 May 20;176 Suppl:S84–96.
69. Castro CM, Wilcox S, O'Sullivan P, Baumann K, King AC. An exercise program for women who are caring for relatives with dementia. *Psychosom Med.* 2002 May-Jun;64(3):458–68.
70. Paladini AC, Marder M, Viola H, Wolfman C, Wasowski C, Medina JH. Flavonoids and the central nervous system: from forgotten factors to potent anxiolytic compounds. *J Pharm Pharmacol* 1999 May;51(5):519–26.
71. Viola H, Wolfman C, Levi de Stein M, Wasowski C, Pena C, Medina JH, Paladini AC. Isolation of pharmacologically active benzodiazepine receptor ligands from Tilia tomentosa (Tiliaceae). J Ethnopharmacol 1994 Aug; 44(1):47–53.
72. Butterweck V, Nishibe S, Sasaki T, Uchida M. Antidepressant effects of apocynum venetum leaves in a forced swimming test. *Biol Pharm Bull.* 2001 Jul;24(7):848–51.
73. Gaby A. Can depressed people benefit from folic acid supplementation? *Townsend Letter for Doctors and Patients.* 2001 Jan.
74. Thompson MB, Coppens NM. The effects of guided imagery on anxiety levels and movement of clients undergoing magnetic resonance imaging. *Holist Nurs Pract.* 1994 Jan;8(2):59–69.
75. Holden-Lund C. Effects of relaxation with guided imagery on surgical stress and wound healing. *Res Nurs Health.* 1988 Aug;11(4):235–44.
76. Speck BJ. The effect of guided imagery upon first semester nursing students performing their first injections. *J Nurs Educ.* 1990 Oct;29(8): 346–50.
77. Houldin AD, McCorkle R, Lowery BJ. Relaxation training and psychoimmunological status of bereaved spouses. A pilot study. *Cancer Nurs.* 1993 Feb;16(1):47–52.
78. McKinney CH, Antoni MH, Kumar M, Tims FC, McCabe PM. Effects of guided imagery and music (GIM) therapy on mood and cortisol in healthy adults. *Health Psychol.* 1997 Jul;16(4):390–400.
79. Rees BL. Effect of relaxation with guided imagery on anxiety, depression, and self-esteem in primiparas. *J Holist Nurs.* 1995 Sep;13(3):255 67.

References

80. Eller LS. Guided imagery interventions for symptom management. *Annu Rev Nurs Res.* 1999;17:57–84.

81. Burns DS. The effect of the bonny method of guided imagery and music on the mood and life quality of cancer patients. *J Music Ther.* 2001 Spring;38(1):51–65.

82. Leja AM. Using guided imagery to combat postsurgical depression. *J Gerontol Nurs.* 1989 Apr;15(4):7–11.

83. Liske E, Hanggi W, Henneicke-von Zepelin HH, Boblitz N, Wustenberg P, Rahlfs VW. Physiological investigation of a unique extract of black cohosh (Cimicifugae racemosae rhizoma): a 6–month clinical study demonstrates no systemic estrogenic effect. *J Womens Health Gend Based Med.* 2002 Mar;11(2):163–74.

84. Satyan KS, Jaiswal AK, Ghosal S, Bhattacharya SK. Anxiolytic activity of ginkgolic acid conjugates from Indian Ginkgo biloba. *Psychopharmacology (Berl)* 1998 Mar;136(2):148–52.

85. Bradwejn J, Zhou Y, Koszycki D, Shlik J. A double-blind, placebo-controlled study on the effects of Gotu Kola (Centella asiatica) on acoustic startle response in healthy subjects. *J Clin Psychopharmacol.* 2000 Dec;20(6):680–4.

86. Malsch U, Kieser M. Efficacy of kava-kava in the treatment of non-psychotic anxiety, following pretreatment with benzodiazepines. *Psychopharmacology (Berl)* 2001 Sep;157(3):277–83.

87. Watkins LL, Connor KM, Davidson JR. Effect of kava extract on vagal cardiac control in generalized anxiety disorder: preliminary findings. *J Psychopharmacol* 2001 Dec;15(4):283–6.

88. Wheatley D. Kava and valerian in the treatment of stress-induced insomnia. *Phytother Res.* 2001 Sep;15(6):549–51.

89. Pittler MH, Edzard E. Kava extract for treating anxiety. *Cochrane Database Syst Rev* 2001;(4):CD003383.

90. Grunze H, Langosch J, Schirrmacher K, Bingmann D, Von Wegerer J, Walden J. Kava pyrones exert effects on neuronal transmission and trans-membraneous cation currents similar to established mood stabilizers—a review. *Prog Neuropsychopharmacol Biol Psychiatry* 2001 Nov;25(8): 1555–70.

91. Gerhard U, Linnenbrink N, Georghiadou C, Hobi V. Vigilance-decreasing effects of 2 plant-derived sedatives. *Schweiz Rundsch Med Prax.* 1996 Apr 9;85(15):473–81.

References

92. Sakamoto T, Mitani Y, Nakajima K. Psychotropic effects of Japanese valerian root extract. *Chem Pharm Bull (Tokyo)* 1992 Mar;40(3):758–61.

93. Cropley M, Cave Z, Ellis J, Middleton RW. Effect of kava and valerian on human physiological and psychological responses to mental stress assessed under laboratory conditions. *Phytother Res* 2002 Feb;16(1):23–7.

94. Alibeu JP, Jobert J. Aconite in homeopathic relief of post-operative pain and agitation in children. *Pediatrie*. 1990;45(7–8):465–6.

95. Yapko M. Hypnosis in treating symptoms and risk factors of major depression. *Am J Clin Hypn*. 2001 Oct;44(2):97–108.

96. Palan BM, Lakhani JD. Converting the "threat" into a "challenge": a case of stress-related hemoptysis managed with hypnosis. *Am J Clin Hypn*. 1991 Apr;33(4):241–7.

97. Gruzelier J, Smith F, Nagy A, Henderson D. Cellular and humoral immunity, mood and exam stress: the influences of self-hypnosis and personality predictors. *Int J Psychophysiol*. 2001 Aug;42(1):55–71.

98. Palatnik A, Frolov K, Fux M, Benjamin J. Double-blind, controlled, crossover trial of inositol versus fluvoxamine for the treatment of panic disorder. *J Clin Psychopharmacol*. 2001 Jun;21(3):335–9.

99. Benjamin J, Agam G, Levine J, Bersudsky Y, Kofman O, Belmaker RH. Inositol treatment in psychiatry. *Psychopharmacol Bull*. 1995;31(1):167–75.

100. Takahashi K, Iwase M, Yamashita K, Tatsumoto Y, Ue H, Kuratsune H, Shimizu A, Takeda M. The elevation of natural killer cell activity induced by laughter in a crossover designed study. *Int J Mol Med*. 2001 Dec;8(6):645–50.

101. Oren DA, Wisner KL, Spinelli M, Epperson CN, Peindl KS, Terman JS, Terman M. An open trial of morning light therapy for treatment of antepartum depression. *Am J Psychiatry*. 2002 Apr;159(4):666–9.

102. Lam RW, Carter D, Misri S, Kuan AJ, Yatham LN, Zis AP. A controlled study of light therapy in women with late luteal phase dysphoric disorder. *Psychiatry Res*. 1999 Jun 30;86(3):185–92.

103. Thorell LH, Kjellman B, Arned M, Lindwall-Sundel K, Walinder J, Wetterberg L. Light treatment of seasonal affective disorder in combination with citalopram or placebo with 1–year follow-up. *Int Clin Psychopharmacol*. 1999 May;14 Suppl 2:S7–11.

104. Leppamaki SJ, Partonen TT, Hurme J, Haukka JK, Lonnqvist JK. Randomized trial of the efficacy of bright-light exposure and aerobic exercise

on depressive symptoms and serum lipids. *J Clin Psychiatry.* 2002 Apr; 63(4):316–21.

105. Haffmans PM, Sival RC, Lucius SA, Cats Q, van Gelder L. Bright light therapy and melatonin in motor restless behaviour in dementia: a placebo-controlled study. *Int J Geriatr Psychiatry.* 2001 Jan;16(1):106–10.

106. Janicak PG, Dowd SM, Martis B, Alam D, Beedle D, Krasuski J, Strong MJ, Sharma R, Rosen C, Viana M. Repetitive transcranial magnetic stimulation versus electroconvulsive therapy for major depression: preliminary results of a randomized trial. *Biol Psychiatry.* 2002 Apr 15;51(8):659–67.

107. Hoffman RE, Cavus I. Slow transcranial magnetic stimulation, long-term depotentiation, and brain hyperexcitability disorders. *Am J Psychiatry.* 2002 Jul;159(7):1093–102.

108. McNamara B, Ray JL, Arthurs OJ, Boniface S.Transcranial magnetic stimulation for depression and other psychiatric disorders. *Psychol Med.* 2001 Oct;31(7):1141–6.

109. Moser DJ, Jorge RE, Manes F, Paradiso S, Benjamin ML, Robinson RG. Improved executive functioning following repetitive transcranial magnetic stimulation. *Neurology.* 2002 Apr 23;58(8):1288–90.

110. Smesny S, Volz HP, Liepert J, Tauber R, Hochstetter A, Sauer H.Repetitive transcranial magnetic stimulation (rTMS) in the acute and long-term therapy of refractory depression—a case report. *Nervenarzt.* 2001 Sep; 72(9):734–8.

111. Reibel DK, Greeson JM, Brainard GC, Rosenzweig S. Mindfulness-based stress reduction and health-related quality of life in a heterogeneous patient population. *Gen Hosp Psychiatry.* 2001 Jul-Aug;23(4):183–92.

112. Speca M, Carlson LE, Goodey E, Angen M. A randomized, wait-list controlled clinical trial: the effect of a mindfulness meditation-based stress reduction program on mood and symptoms of stress in cancer outpatients. *Psychosom Med.* 2000 Sep-Oct;62(5):613–22.

113. Shapiro SL, Schwartz GE, Bonner G. Effects of mindfulness-based stress reduction on medical and premedical students. *J Behav Med.* 1998 Dec;21(6):581–99.

114. Citera G, Arias MA, Maldonado-Cocco JA, Lazaro MA, Rosemffet MG, Brusco LI, Scheines EJ, Cardinalli DP. The effect of melatonin in patients with fibromyalgia: a pilot study. *Clin Rheumatol.* 2000;19(1):9–13.

115. Garfinkel D, Zisapel N, Wainstein J, Laudon M. Facilitation of benzodi-

References

azepine discontinuation by melatonin: a new clinical approach. *Arch Intern Med*. 1999 Nov 8;159(20):2456–60.

116. Guidi L, Tricerri A, Frasca D, Vangeli M, Errani AR, Bartoloni C. Psychoneuroimmunology and aging. *Gerontology*. 1998;44(5):247–61.

117. Kiecolt-Glaser JK, McGuire L, Robles TF, Glaser R. Emotions, morbidity, and mortality: new perspectives from psychoneuroimmunology. *Annu Rev Psychol*. 2002;53:83–107.

118. Sali A. Psychoneuroimmunology. Fact or fiction? *Aust Fam Physician*. 1997 Nov;26(11):1291–4, 1296–9.

119. Berk M, Wadee AA, Kuschke RH, O'Neill-Kerr A. Acute phase proteins in major depression. *J Psychosom Res*. 1997 Nov;43(5):529–34.

120. Raison CL, Miller AH. The neuroimmunology of stress and depression. *Semin Clin Neuropsychiatry*. 2001 Oct;6(4):277–94.

121. Hashiro M, Okumura M. The relationship between the psychological and immunological state in patients with atopic dermatitis. *J Dermatol Sci*. 1998 Mar;16(3):231–5.

122. Wada H. Problems and strategies in the treatment of mental disorders in elderly patients with physical illness. *Nippon Ronen Igakkai Zasshi*. 2000 Nov;37(11):885–8.

123. Barrows KA, Jacobs BP. Mind-body medicine. An introduction and review of the literature. *Med Clin North Am* 2002 Jan;86(1):11–31.

124. Hamel WJ. The effects of music intervention on anxiety in the patient waiting for cardiac catheterization. *Intensive Crit Care Nurs*. 2001 Oct;17(5):279–85.

125. Renzi C, Peticca L, Pescatori M. The use of relaxation techniques in the perioperative management of proctological patients: preliminary results. *Int J Colorectal Dis*. 2000 Nov;15(5–6):313–6.

126. Myskja A, Lindbaek M. Examples of the use of music in clinical medicine. *Tidsskr Nor Laegeforen*. 2000 Apr 10;120(10):1186–90.

127. Metzger JY, Berthou V, Perrin P, Sichel JP. Phototherapy: clinical and therapeutic evaluation of a 2–year experience. *Encephale*. 1998 Sep-Oct; 24(5):480–5.

128. Carbonell DM, Parteleno-Barehmi C. Psychodrama groups for girls coping with trauma. *Int J Group Psychother*. 1999 Jul;49(3):285–306.

129. Soo S, Moayyedi P, Deeks J, Delaney B, Lewis M, Forman D. Psychological interventions for non-ulcer dyspepsia. *Cochrane Database Syst Rev*.

References

2001;(4): CD002301.

130. Satya AJ. Stress management for patient and physician. *J Indian Med Assoc*. 2001 Feb;99(2):90–2.

131. Koenig HG. Religion and medicine III: developing a theoretical model. *Int J Psychiatry Med*. 2001;31(2):199–216.

132. Jones ED, Beck-Little R. The use of reminiscence therapy for the treatment of depression in rural-dwelling older adults. *Issues Ment Health Nurs*. 2002 Apr;23(3):279–90.

133. Turner JG, Clark AJ, Gauthier DK, Williams M. The effect of therapeutic touch on pain and anxiety in burn patients. *J Adv Nurs*. 1998 Jul;28(1):10–20.

134. Giasson M, Bouchard L. Effect of therapeutic touch on the well-being of persons with terminal cancer. *J Holist Nurs*. 1998 Sep;16(3):383–98.

135. Kiernan J. The experience of Therapeutic Touch in the lives of five postpartum women. *MCN Am J Matern Child Nurs*. 2002 Jan-Feb;27(1):47–53.

136. Hughes PP, Meize-Grochowski R, Harris CN. Therapeutic touch with adolescent psychiatric patients. *J Holist Nurs*. 1996 Mar;14(1):6–23.

137. Comazzi AM, Nielsen NP, Zizolfi S, Dioguardi N. Neurotic and depressive status related to organic pathology in patients in thermal therapy. *Minerva Med*. 1991 Jul-Aug;82(7–8):463–75.

138. Smidt LJ, Cremin FM, Grivetti LE, Clifford AJ. Influence of thiamin supplementation on the health and general well-being of an elderly Irish population with marginal thiamin deficiency. *J Gerontol*. 1991 Jan;46(1): M16–22.

139. Sacks W, Esser AH, Feitel B, Abbott K. Acetazolamide and thiamine: an ancillary therapy for chronic mental illness. *Psychiatry Res*. 1989 Jun;28(3):279–88.

140. Meins W, Muller-Thomsen T, Meier-Baumgartner HP. Subnormal serum vitamin B12 and behavioural and psychological symptoms in Alzheimer's disease. *Int J Geriatr Psychiatry*. 2000 May;15(5):415–8.